MERCER UNIVERSITY MAIN LIBRARY

Genetic Studies in Affective Disorders

An Einstein Psychiatry Publication

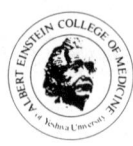

Publication Series of the Department of Psychiatry
Albert Einstein College of Medicine of Yeshiva University
New York, NY

Editor-in-Chief Herman M. van Praag, M.D., Ph.D.
Associate Editor Demitri Papolos, M.D.

Editorial Board

Gregory Asnis, M.D.
Jeffrey Bedell, Ph.D.
Evan Imber Black, Ph.D.
Anne Etgen, Ph.D.
Eliot L. Gardner, Ph.D.
T. Byram Karasu, M.D.
Martin M. Katz, Ph.D.
John M. Kane, M.D.

Jean Pierre Lindenmayer, M.D.
Arnie Merriam, M.D.
Fred Pine, Ph.D.
Robert Plutchik, Ph.D.
David Preven, M.D.
Peter Stastny, M.D.
Scott Wetzler, Ph.D.
Stephen Zukin, M.D.

1. CONTEMPORARY APPROACHES TO PSYCHOLOGICAL ASSESSMENT
   Edited by Scott Wetzler, Ph.D. & Martin M. Katz, Ph.D.

2. COMPUTER APPLICATIONS IN PSYCHIATRY AND PSYCHOLOGY
   Edited by David Baskin, Ph.D.

3. VIOLENCE AND SUICIDALITY: PERSPECTIVES IN CLINICAL
   AND PSYCHOBIOLOGICAL RESEARCH
   *Edited by Herman M. van Praag, M.D., Ph.D.,
   Robert Plutchik, Ph.D., & Alan Apter, M.D.*

4. THE ROLE OF SEROTONIN IN PSYCHIATRIC DISORDERS
   *Edited by Serena-Lynn Brown, M.D., Ph.D.
   & Herman M. van Praag, M.D., Ph.D.*

5. POSITIVE AND NEGATIVE SYNDROMES IN SCHIZOPHRENIA:
   ASSESSMENT AND RESEARCH
   by Stanley R. Kay, Ph.D.

6. NEW BIOLOGICAL VISTAS ON SCHIZOPHRENIA
   *Edited by Jean-Pierre Lindenmayer, M.D.
   & Stanley R. Kay, Ph.D.*

7. "MAKE-BELIEVES" IN PSYCHIATRY, OR THE PERILS OF PROGRESS
   by Herman M. van Praag, M.D., Ph.D.

8. GENETIC STUDIES IN AFFECTIVE DISORDERS: BASIC METHODS,
   CURRENT DIRECTIONS, AND CRITICAL RESEARCH ISSUES
   *Edited by Demitri F. Papolos, M.D.
   & Herbert M. Lachman, M.D.*

Einstein Psychiatry Publication No. 8

Genetic Studies in Affective Disorders

Overview of Basic Methods, Current Directions, and Critical Research Issues

Edited by

DEMITRI F. PAPOLOS
HERBERT M. LACHMAN

A Wiley-Interscience Publication
John Wiley & Sons, Inc.

New York • Chichester • Brisbane • Toronto • Singapore

This text is printed on acid-free paper.

Copyright © 1994 by John Wiley & Sons, Inc.

All rights reserved. Published simultaneously in Canada.

Reproduction or translation of any part of this work beyond that permitted by Section 107 or 108 of the 1976 United States Copyright Act without the permission of the copyright owner is unlawful. Requests for permission or further information should be addressed to the Permissions Department, John Wiley & Sons, Inc., 605 Third Avenue, New York, NY 10158-0012.

This publication is designed to provide accurate and authoritative information in regard to the subject matter covered. It is sold with the understanding that the publisher is not engaged in rendering legal, accounting, or other professional services. If legal advice or other expert assistance is required, the services of a competent professional person should be sought. *From a Declaration of Principles jointly adopted by a Committee of the American Bar Association and a Committee of Publishers.*

Library of Congress Cataloging in Publication Data:

Genetic studies in affective disorders : overview of basic methods, current directions, and critical research issues / edited by Demitri F. Papolos, Herbert M. Lachman.
    p.   cm. — (Publication series of the Department of Psychiatry Albert Einstein College of Medicine of Yeshiva University ; 8)
  Includes index.
  ISBN 0-471-00075-2 (cloth)
  1. Affective disorders—Genetic aspects. I. Papolos, Demitri F. II. Lachman, Herbert M. III. Series.
RC537.G46 1994
616.89'5042—dc20   93-6161

Printed in the United States of America

10 9 8 7 6 5 4 3 2 1

Contributors

Miron Baron, M.D., Professor of Clinical Psychiatry, College of Physicians and Surgeons of Columbia University, New York, New York.

Emmeline Edwards, Ph.D., Associate Professor, Department of Pharmacology and Toxicology, University of Maryland at Baltimore, Baltimore, Maryland.

Janice A. Egeland, Ph.D., Professor of Psychiatry and Epidemiology, Department of Psychiatry, University of Miami, Miami, Florida.

Jean Endicott, Ph.D., Professor of Clinical Psychology, Department of Psychiatry, College of Physicians and Surgeons of Columbia University, New York, New York.

Stephen V. Faraone, Ph.D., at the Massachusetts Mental Health Center, Boston, and Assistant Professor Department of Psychiatry, Harvard Medical School; Brockton/West Roxbury VA Medical Center, Brockton, Massachusetts.

Shalom Feinberg, M.D., Assistant Clinical Professor of Psychiatry, Albert Einstein College of Medicine/Montefiore Medical Center, Bronx, New York; Attending Psychiatrist, The Holliswood Hospital, Holliswood, New York.

Robin R. Green, M.A., Research Associate, Department of Psychiatry, Brockton/West Roxbury VA Medical Center, Brockton, Massachusetts.

Fritz A. Henn, Ph.D., M.D., Professor and Chairman, Department of Psychiatry, State University of New York at Stony Brook, Stony Brook, New York.

Herbert M. Lachman, M.D., Associate Professor, Department of Medicine and Psychiatry, Albert Einstein College of Medicine/Montefiore Medical Center, Bronx, New York.

Julien Mendlewicz, M.D., Ph.D., Chairman Department of Psychiatry, Erasme Hospital, Free University of Brussels, Brussels, Belgium.

Demitri F. Papolos, M.D., Assistant Professor, Department of Psychiatry, Albert Einstein College of Medicine/Montefiore Medical Center, Bronx, New York.

David L. Pauls, Ph.D., Associate Professor of Human Genetics, Yale University Child Study Center, New Haven, Connecticut.

Ming T. Tsuang, M.D., Ph.D., Stanley Cobb Professor of Psychiatry, Director of Psychiatric Epidemiology, Harvard Schools of Medicine and Public Health, Boston, Massachusetts and Head, Department of Psychiatry, Harvard Medical School at the Massachusetts Mental Health Center, and Brockton/West Roxbury VA Medical Center, Brockton, Massachusetts.

A Note on the Series

Psychiatry is in a state of flux. The excitement springs in part from internal changes, such as the development and official acceptance (at least in the United States) of an operationalized, multi-axial classification system of behavioral disorders (the DSM-III), the increasing sophistication of methods to measure abnormal human behavior, and the impressive expansion of biological and psychological treatment modalities. Exciting developments are also taking place in fields relating to psychiatry; in molecular (brain) biology, genetics, brain imaging, drug development, epidemiology, experimental psychology, to mention only a few striking examples.

More generally speaking, psychiatry is moving, still relatively slowly, but irresistibly from a more philosophical, contemplative orientation to that of an empirical science. From the 1950s on, biological psychiatry has been a major catalyst of that process. It provided the mother discipline with a third cornerstone, that is, neurobiology, the other two being psychology and medical sociology. In addition, it forced the profession into the direction of standardization of diagnoses and of assessment of abnormal behavior. Biological psychiatry provided psychiatry not only with a new basic science and with new treatment modalities, but also with the tools, the methodology, and the mentality to operate within the confines of an empirical science, the only framework in which a medical discipline can survive.

In other fields of psychiatry, too, one discerns a gradual trend towards scientification. Psychological treatment techniques are standardized and manuals developed to make these skills more easily transferable. Methods registering treatment outcome—traditionally used in the behavioral/cognitive field—are now more and more requested and, hence, developed for dynamic forms of psychotherapy as well. Social and community psychiatry, until the 1960s were more firmly rooted in humanitarian ideals and social awareness than in empirical studies, profited greatly from its liaison with the social sciences and the expansion of psychiatric epidemiology.

Let there be no misunderstanding. Empiricism does *not imply* that it is only the measurable that counts. Psychiatry would be mutilated if it would neglect that which cannot be captured by numbers. It *does imply* that what is measurable should be measured. Progress in psychiatry is dependent on ideas and on experiment. Their linkage is inseparable.

This Series, published under the auspices of the Department of Psychiatry of the Albert Einstein College of Medicine, Montefiore Medical Center, is meant to keep track of important developments in our profession, to summarize what has been achieved in particular fields, and to bring together the viewpoints obtained from disparate vantage points—in short, to capture some of the ongoing excitement in modern psychiatry, both in its clinical and experimental dimensions. The Department of Psychiatry at Albert Einstein College of Medicine hosts the Series, but naturally welcomes contributions from others.

Bernie Mazel originally generated the idea for the series—an ambitious plan which we all felt was worthy of pursuit. The edifice of psychiatry is impressive, but still somewhat flawed in its foundations. May this Series contribute to consolidation of its infrastructure.

—HERMAN M. VAN PRAAG, M.D., PH.D.
Professor and Chairman
Academic Psychiatric Center
University of Limburg
Maastricht
The Netherlands

Preface

For both of us, the publication of this volume represents a personal milestone on a long path that began with direct experience of the profound impact of manic-depressive illness, an appreciation of the havoc that it has brought to countless afflicted individuals, and the knowledge that the techniques to search for the gene(s) that are responsible for this condition are now at hand.

The behavioral disturbances and family disruption that manic depression brings in its wake will likely yield to the intellectual and technical advances to be made over the next decade. The path towards this goal has been most recently illuminated by the work of many of the contributors to this volume, and the early history of this unusual enterprise is put forth in these pages.

To date, there has been no single source available within the psychiatric literature that brings together in one place a description of contemporary genetic linkage studies, current methodologies; diagnostic, statistical and molecular, in the study of bipolar disorder. The impetus for this book has been to provide a resource for psychiatrists, residents and mental health professionals with little or no background in molecular genetics. Moreover, we hope that it will offer up-to-date information to clinicians who are increasingly called upon by patients and families to provide information about the genetic nature and potential heritability of these conditions.

We would like to express our gratitude to Herman M. van Pragg, M.D., PhD., whose vision and support was instrumental in establishing the Program in Behavioral Genetics at Albert Einstein College of Medicine, and to Byram Karasu, M.D. who has continued that support in his new role as Chairman of the Department of Psychiatry. A special thanks to our fine editor at John Wiley & Sons, Herb Reich, and to the talented folks at Publications Development Company who wrestled with a sometimes untidy manuscript.

DEMITRI F. PAPOLOS
HERBERT M. LACHMAN

Contents

Introduction   xiii

PART I. BASIC METHODS, CURRENT DIRECTIONS, AND CRITICAL RESEARCH ISSUES IN LINKAGE STUDIES

1. Genetic Epidemiology of Mood Disorders   3
   MING T. TSUANG,
   STEPHEN V. FARAONE, AND
   ROBIN R. GREEN

2. Diagnostic Issues in Pedigree Assessment   28
   JEAN ENDICOTT AND
   MIRON BARON

3. Basic Principles in Linkage Analysis   46
   HERBERT M. LACHMAN

4. An Epidemiologic and Genetic Study of Affective Disorders among the Old Order Amish   70
   JANICE A. EGELAND

5. Genetic Linkage Studies in Psychiatry: *Strengths and Weaknesses*   91
   DAVID L. PAULS

6. Molecular Genetic Studies in Affective Illness   105
   JULIEN MENDLEWIC

PART II. CLINICAL ASPECTS OF THE GENETIC STUDIES

7. The Family Psychoeducational Approach: *Rationale for a Multigenerational Treatment Modality for the Major Affective Disorders*   119

    DEMITRI F. PAPOLOS

8. Genetic Counseling Issues in Affective Disorders: *The Orthodox Jewish Community*   146

    SHALOM FEINBERG

PART III. ANIMAL MODELS AND IN VITRO SYSTEMS: FUTURE DIRECTIONS

9. Animal Models in the Study of Genetic Factors in Human Psychopathology   177

    FRITZ A. HENN AND
    EMMELINE EDWARDS

10. Lithium's Effect on Gene Expression: *Implications for the Pathogenesis of Mood Disorders*   193

    HERBERT M. LACHMAN

Author Index   219

Subject Index   230

Introduction

Mood disorders are the "common cold" of major psychiatric illnesses. The President's Commission on Mental Health estimates that in the United States over 20 million people will develop a mood disorder during their lifetime. At any given time, 3 to 5% of the population will be suffering from a major depressive or manic episode. One in five families will directly feel their disorder's impact. Those who have a manic-depressive illness will alternate between periods of superactivity, manic elation, and grandiose schemes and periods of despondency, immobility, guilt, and the inability to experience pleasure. Those who suffer recurrent severe depression without periods of mania or hypomania have unipolar or nonbipolar major depression. The psychiatric profession groups both types of mood disturbances under the rubric "major affective disorders" or mood disorders.

The similar rates of mood disorders in every race, culture, and geographic location have bolstered the suspicion that manic-depressive disorder has a biological and, very probably, a genetic basis. The acceptance of genetics as an important factor in mental illness has come slowly. Twenty years ago, the idea of a genetic influence on complex human behavior was anathema to many behavioral scientists, and yet, well before that time, the pioneers of modern psychiatry in Europe and the United States had grasped the importance of genetics and had undertaken family and epidemiologic studies as an integral part of their research. Over the past half century, numerous twin, adoption, and family studies have suggested that genetic factors are important in the etiology of mood disorders.

The most convincing level of genetic evidence, however, involves proof of linkage to a known genetic marker—two traits segregating together in families because the genes that determine the two traits are located near one another on a chromosome. It is at this stage that the complexities of psychiatric disorders become serious obstacles, because the simple genetic models—autosomal, X-linked dominant, and recessive—must be modified to account for nongenetic factors. Confounding factors such as age-related penetrance, variable presentations of illness within the same families, and lack of consensus diagnoses precluded the development of a working genetic model until 1985. But with the use of modern statistical techniques such as linkage analysis, clear evidence has emerged showing that familial patterns are consistent with specific genetic models.

In the past 10 years, recombinant DNA techniques have enabled researches to isolate and clone the aberrant genes in a variety of genetic disorders, including cystic fibrosis, neurofibromatosis, and Huntington's disease. Recently, linkage studies using recombinant DNA methodology have provided an innovative strategy for elucidating the role of genetic factors in the etiology of psychiatric disorders and have presented a unique opportunity to examine hypotheses about genetic transmission. This method requires that a genetic marker be linked to and travel in close company with the abnormal gene locus on the same chromosome. One type of DNA marker used in linkage studies is restriction fragment length polymorphisms (RFLPs). These natural, random mutations in human DNA provide the signposts by which unique variations among individuals can be tracked directly within the genome. The identification of numerous RFLP markers located on every human chromosome has led to the development of a linkage map of the human genome, which theoretically affords the possibility of mapping virtually any inherited disorder to a particular location on a chromosome.

Linkage analysis is a powerful strategy for identifying the chromosomal location of a disorder caused by a single gene that has its effect regardless of environmental or genetic background, as in Huntington's disease. Unfortunately, this may not be the case for psychiatric disorders. The problem of genetic heterogeneity, where several genes, possibly on different chromosomes, are responsible for producing the same or similar phenotypes in a sample of families, remains one of the most serious obstacles to the current research effort. In addition, biological or environmental factors that interact with the genetic predisposition may prevent the expression of the illness, contributing to a greater difficulty in identifying the target gene through classical linkage analysis. In addition to using random RFLPs to search the human genome of affected families, candidate genes, whose protein products and location in the brain bear some relationship to a described model of illness, are being sought and used as specific probes.

This book begins with a chapter by Dr. Ming Tsuang and colleagues that explores the history and development of modern genetic epidemiologic studies of the major affective disorders, and it then focuses on studies among the Old Order Amish of Lancaster, PA, in which an autosomal dominant pattern of inheritance has been found, and on Belgian pedigrees in whom manic depressive illness has been found to be linked to the X chromosome. The chapters by Drs. Janice Egeland and Julien Mendlewicz, pioneers in family and pedigree studies, not only introduce the reader to the primary research findings, but offer a rich overview in their respective areas of interest and point to new directions that the research is likely to follow over the coming years.

The significant advances in molecular biological techniques, including gene mapping, polymorphism detection, and the candidate gene approach as they are applied to genetic studies of inherited psychiatric disorders, are detailed by Dr. Herb Lachman in a straightforward and lucid manner that can be easily grasped by readers with a fundamental knowledge of genetics and biology.

It is our intent that readers also gain a clearer understanding of the impact of clinical diagnostic issues on the evidence for linkage, as well as of diagnostic issues that commonly arise in pedigree assessment and ascertainment. To this end, the chapter by Drs. Jean Endicott and Miron Baron amply elucidates basic issues in RFLP linkage and association studies, including methods of pedigree ascertainment and statistical methods used in the analyses of data. Employing a simulation model, Dr. David Pauls painlessly walks the reader through a basic tutorial designed to elucidate the often intimidating statistical approaches to lod ($\log_{10}$ odds ratio) score determination, while clearly describing the strengths and weaknesses of linkage analysis as it is applied to psychiatric disorders.

A section devoted to the clinical aspects of the genetic studies addresses a number of practical questions: How does the information about the inheritance patterns of these conditions guide us in our work with patients and their families? How might the new knowledge gained from epidemiologic and genetic studies expand and shape our clinical view and contribute to the development of innovative methods of treatment? What are the psychological and ethical considerations of genetic counseling? The chapters by Drs. Demitri Papolos and Shalom Feinberg attempt to address these complex issues, while providing useful and timely information to clinicians involved in the treatment of patients with recurrent mood disorders.

The final section on animal models and in vitro systems includes a chapter by Drs. Fritz Henn and Emmeline Edwards that describes the development of an animal model for depression that uses the paradigm of learned helplessness and provides the opportunity to examine the interplay between environmental stressors and genetic susceptibility that produces depression within a neurobiolgical framework. Finally, Dr. Lachman examines studies on the molecular basis of lithium action, in particular, the effect of lithium salts on the regulation of gene expression in neuronal cells.

The text is directed toward psychiatric residents, clinical and academic psychiatrists, psychologists, and social workers, as well as medical students and health care workers interested in developing a greater knowledge of recent molecular genetic approaches as they are applied to inherited behavioral disorders.

DEMITRI F. PAPOLOS, M.D.
HERBERT M. LACHMAN, M.D.
Editors

PART I
Basic Methods, Current Directions, and Critical Research Issues in Linkage Studies

1

Genetic Epidemiology of Mood Disorders

MING T. TSUANG,
STEPHEN V. FARAONE, AND
ROBIN R. GREEN

Genetic epidemiologic investigation is a relatively recent discipline that has been found to be useful in researching psychiatric disorders. It has its roots in epidemiology and genetics. Epidemiologists have attempted to quantify and understand rates of illness and to explain the clustering of cases in circumscribed geographical regions. However, they usually have not studied the influence of genetic diversity and have tended to search for environmental risk factors and causes for diseases. Geneticists, on the other hand, have tended to focus primarily on genetic mechanisms for diseases. The experimental genetic study of plants and animals has made great strides by manipulating genetic strains while holding the environment constant. Genetic epidemiology combines these two traditions of epidemiology and genetics by taking into account environmental as well as genetic risk factors of disease. Morton (1982) defines the discipline as "a science that deals with the cause, distribution, and control of disease in groups of relatives and with the inherited causes of disease in populations."

Preparation of this article was supported in part by the Veterans Administration's Medical Research and Health Services Research and Development Programs and National Institute of Mental Health Grants 1 R01MH41879-01, 5 U01 MH46318-02, and R37MH43518-01. Requests for reprints should be sent to Ming T. Tsuang, M.D., Department of Psychiatry, Harvard Medical School at the Massachusetts Mental Health Center, 74 Fenwood Rd., Boston, MA 02115.

Focusing principally on the distribution of illness within families, genetic epidemiologic studies attempt to separate the effects and interactions of genes and environment. Thus, genetic epidemiologic studies are particularly valuable in the investigation of psychiatric disorders, many of which are caused by the fusion of genetic and environmental factors. In practice, the genetic epidemiologic investigation of disorders attempts to answer the following four questions: Is the disorder familial? What are the relative contributions of genetic and environmental factors to the disease etiology? What is the mode of transmission in families? What are the genetic and environmental mechanisms of the disease? In this chapter, we briefly review the answers to these questions for the genetics of mood disorders. A more detailed presentation is provided by Tsuang and Faraone (1990).

ARE MOOD DISORDERS FAMILIAL?

If genes cause mood disorders, then the relatives of mood disordered patients should be at greater risk for the illness than the relatives of nonpatients. In genetic epidemiology, we use the term *proband* to designate patients and nonpatients who are initially identified for a research study. According to the laws of genetic inheritance, the risk to relatives of probands is a function of the number of genes they share with the proband. The relatives who share 50% of their genes with the proband are parents, children, and siblings (first-degree relatives). Relatives who share only 25% of the genes with the proband are grandparents, uncles, aunts, nephews, and nieces (second-degree relatives). Under a genetic hypothesis, first-degree relatives of mood-disordered probands are at a higher risk for mood disorders than are second-degree relatives because the former share a higher percentage of genes (50%) than the latter. In short, the hypothesis that genes predispose to illness predicts that the relatives of mood-disordered probands are at a greater risk for the disorder than are the relatives of control probands, and that the risk to relatives of ill probands decreases based on the percentage of genes they share. That is, individuals who are less closely related genetically to an ill proband will be at lower risk for the disorder.

Because family studies are relatively easy to implement, they are useful in the initial stages of psychiatric genetic research. However, although a genetic hypothesis predicts that a disorder will be familial, familiality can occur for other reasons. Most notably, family members share a common culture and a common environment. Since the similarity of these factors tends to increase as the degree of the relationship decreases, familial–environmental factors may confound genetic relationships. For example, if cigarette smoking is a habit that children learn from parents, then one might observe that smoking-related disorders run in families. In this case, familial transmission is due primarily to relatives' sharing a common environmental pathogen. Possible sources of cultural and environmental transmission include bacteria, viruses, learned responses to stress, and cultural differences in emotional expression. Thus, the interpretation of familial transmission as genetic must be tentative because a disorder can be familial owing to environmental and cultural factors. In addition, the failure to find familial transmission can strongly suggest that a disorder does not have a substantial genetic component. Ideally, the family study uses double-blind, case-controlled methodology so that the diagnoses of relatives are made independently of the proband's diagnosis. Controlled studies are preferable. However, in the absence of a control group, it is common to compare family study results with population risks from epidemiologic studies.

Epidemiologic Population Studies

Before examining family studies of mood disorders, we will take a broader, epidemiologic view of these disorders. Population-based epidemiologic studies are useful in this regard because they provide a context in which family study data can be interpreted. Early epidemiologic studies of "manic-depressive psychosis," performed from 1938 to 1952, found the risk for the illness in the general population to range from 0.4% to 1.7%. The mean risk was 0.7% (Tsuang & Faraone, 1990). Table 1–1 presents the results of more recent epidemiologic studies of bipolar disorder. These studies examine the risk of bipolar disorder among individuals randomly selected from a specified catchment area. As Table 1–1 indicates, the risk of bipolar disorder ranges

TABLE 1-1
Percent Risk for Bipolar Disorder among General Population Samples

Study	Percent Risk
Fremming (1951)	0.6
Parsons (1965)	0.9
James & Chapman (1975)	0.2
Smeraldi et al. (1977)	0.1
Helgason (1979)	0.8
Robins et al. (1984)	
New Haven	1.1
Baltimore	0.6
St. Louis	1.1
Weissman et al. (1984)	0.2

Adapted from Tsuang and Faraone (1990).

from 0.1% to 1.1%. Thus, the population risks for bipolar disorder are similar to the risks reported for manic-depressive psychosis from earlier studies.

The risk of unipolar disorder in the general population ranges from 3.4% to 18.0% (Table 1-2). A comparison of Tables 1-1 and 1-2 reveals that unipolar disorder is much more prevalent than bipolar

TABLE 1-2
Percent Risk for Unipolar Disorder among General Population Samples

Study	Percent Risk
Fremming (1951)	16.3
Essen-Moller & Hagnell (1961)	3.4
Helgason (1961)	6.0
Weissman & Meyers (1978)	18.0
Helgason (1979)	12.0
Egeland & Hostetter (1983)	0.5
Robins et al. (1984)	
New Haven	6.7
Baltimore	0.6
St. Louis	5.5
Weissman et al. (1984)	5.9

Adapted from Tsuang and Faraone (1990).

disorder. All of these studies that examine unipolar and bipolar disorders find a greater prevalence of unipolar disorder.

※ Given that the earlier definition of manic-depressive psychosis included both unipolar and bipolar forms of the disorder, it is surprising that the risk for unipolar disorder is so high. One of the possible reasons for this may be that the population risk for mood disorders has increased over time. Several independent investigators have observed an increasing lifetime risk for major depression during the 20th century (Gershon, Hamovit, Guroff, & Nurnberger, 1987; Hagnell, Lanke, Rorsman, & Ojesio, 1982; Klerman, 1976; Klerman et al., 1985; Robins et al., 1984; Srole & Fischer, 1980; Weissman & Myers, 1978). Gershon et al. (1987) and Rice et al. (1987) report a similar trend for bipolar disorder. There are three different effects that may explain the increase in unipolar disorders in this century: a birth cohort effect, a period effect, and an age–period interaction. Klerman et al. (1985) assessed unipolar depression among the 2,289 relatives of 523 probands with mood disorders. The results showed an increasing rate of depression in successive birth cohorts through the 20th century; there was also an earlier age at onset of depression for each successive birth cohort. The lifetime risk of major depression was less than 20% for relatives born before 1910, but rose steadily to more than 60% for relatives born after 1949. We refer to such findings as a "birth cohort effect" because the year of birth is predictive of the risk of depression, with successive birth cohorts being at increased risk for the disorder. However, as Lavori et al. (1986) have pointed out, a cohort effect may also be due to a period effect. A period effect is a factor that affects all individuals for a limited time. An example of a pure period effect given by Lavori et al. is the rate of cancer among the survivors of the atomic bomb explosions in Hiroshima and Nagasaki. This demonstrates that their risk for cancer directly correlates with a distinct period in their lives.

A period effect may be difficult to tease out from a cohort effect when there is an age–period interaction. This occurs when the likelihood of developing the disorder is related to the age of the individual. Thus, although the increasing risk of major depression through the 20th century is consistent with birth cohort effect, it is equally likely that some recent period of time has been associated with an increase in (depressogenic) factors leading to depression that exert stronger effects on younger individuals. The presence of a period effect on the risk for unipolar depression has implications for the genetic study of the disorder. The effect may explain the discrepancies between the early studies of manic-depressive disorder and the more recent studies of bipolar and unipolar disorders since several decades separate the two sets of studies. However, firm conclusions are not possible given that the earlier studies differ in many ways from the later ones. Nevertheless, the rising risk of mood disorders must be taken into account when comparing studies.

Family Studies

Early family studies, were conducted from 1929 to 1954, did not make the distinction between unipolar and bipolar disorders and only report the risk for manic-depressive disorder among relatives of manic-depressive probands (Tsuang & Faraone, 1990). The risk to parents ranged from 3.2% to 23.4%, with a mean of 14.6%. The risk to siblings ranged from 2.7% to 23.0%, with a mean of 10.9%. It is notable that each of the studies finds relatives of mood-disordered probands to be at greater risk for manic-depressive psychosis than the 0.7% general population risk reported by the early epidemiologic studies.

As a whole, the early family studies of major mood disorders consistently suggested that manic-depressive psychosis runs in families. Although the consistency is impressive, these results could be due to the use of research methods that did not include controls for bias. The methods did not involve the use of interviewer blindness or control groups, or the systematic application of age corrections to population and family risk figures. The extent of these problems is difficult to assess because most of these early studies do not provide sufficient details of the methodology used.

With regard to family studies performed during the 1970s and 1980s, an increase in the rigor of scientific research and writing has resulted in reports that allow for a careful look at methodological aspects. In an attempt to address the issue of interviewer bias, these researchers took particular interest in addressing the issue of diagnostic bias. In the ideal family study design, the interviewer is "blind" to the diagnoses of the interviewees' relatives. Also, many of these studies present results separately for unipolar and bipolar subtypes and thus they allow for the examination of the familial association of these two disorders.

Overall, family studies of bipolar probands strongly support the hypothesis that their first-degree relatives are at greater risk of bipolar disorder as compared with the general population. The risk to relatives ranges from a low of 1.2% to a high of 24.9%. All of these values are greater than the general population risk suggested by the epidemiologic studies discussed above. More important, each of the three double-blind, controlled studies found high rates of bipolar disorder among relatives of bipolar probands as compared with relatives of control probands. Conclusions regarding the relationship between unipolar and bipolar subforms are more ambiguous. Studies that limit the definition of unipolar depression to recurrent forms tend to find no familial association. Most of the double-blind, controlled studies find higher rates of unipolar disorder among relatives of bipolar probands in comparison with controls. However, since these studies included nonrecurrent unipolar depression, many of the unipolar cases may be bipolar cases in which the subjects have not yet experienced a first manic episode.

In studying the incidence of unipolar and bipolar disorder in the families of unipolar probands, Perris (1966) reported results from 1203 first-degree relatives of 139 recurrent unipolar probands. Their risk of bipolar disorder was found to be less than 0.5%, much lower than the previously discussed risk for bipolar disorder among relatives of bipolar probands and not much different from what one would expect from general population studies. However, the risk of unipolar disorder among relatives of unipolar probands was 5 to 30 times greater than the risk to relatives of bipolar probands. These results led Perris to suggest that unipolar and bipolar subforms are genetically distinct disorders. Using Perris's criteria for recurrent depression, Smeraldi, Negri, and Melica (1977) found similar results. Trzebiatowska-Trzeciak (1977) also observed independent familial segregation of unipolar and bipolar disorders. Her study included 53 recurrent unipolar probands and their 379 first-degree relatives. The risk of bipolar disorder for first-degree relatives of unipolar probands was only 0.3%, which is well within the population expectation and substantially lower than the risk she found to relatives of bipolar probands. The unipolar risk to unipolar probands (6.3%–8.0%) contrasts sharply with her finding of no unipolar disorder among relatives of bipolar probands.

The double-blind, controlled study of Gershon and colleagues (1982) included 166 first-degree relatives of unipolar probands. Among these relatives, they found a 1.5% risk for bipolar disorder; this was greater than the 0.0% risk for controls, but less than the 4.5% risk for relatives of bipolar probands. The 16.6% risk of unipolar disorder to relatives of unipolar probands was not much greater than the 14.0% risk of unipolar disorder to relatives of bipolar probands, but was nearly three times the risk observed in the control group. These results are similar to those of controlled studies by Tsuang, Winokur, and Crowe (1980) and Gershon, Baron, and Leckman (1975); each of these studies finds strong evidence for a familial component to unipolar disorder and weaker evidence that bipolar disorder is elevated in unipolar families.

Weissman and colleagues (1984) studied psychiatric disorders in 2,003 first-degree relatives of 335 unipolar probands. Probands were diagnosed with structured personal interviews based on the research diagnostic criteria. Relatives were interviewed using the same diagnostic instrument based on the research diagnostic criteria, along with family history evaluations from multiple informants. Approximately 75% of the evaluations of relatives were blind to proband diagnostic status. The researchers assessed a community sample of 82 normal controls with similar diagnostic methodologies. The 8.1% risk of bipolar disorder among relatives of unipolar probands was four times the risk observed in the community. The 18.4% risk of unipolar disorder was three times the risk reported in the community. Thus, consistent with other double-blind, controlled studies, there is evidence for a familial component to unipolar disorder, and some suggestion of a familial coaggregation of unipolar and bipolar disorders.

The study of Endicott and colleagues (1985) included 121 recurrent unipolar probands and their 424 first-degree relatives. The 0.7% risk of bipolar disorder found among the relatives is not much greater than the population expectation and is less than the 2.3% reported for relatives of bipolar probands. The risk of unipolar disorder to relatives of unipolar probands (11.1%) was not much greater than the 8.3% risk to relatives of bipolar probands. The results from the National Institute of Mental Health Collaborative Study of Depression (Andreasen et al.,

1987) found a 0.6% risk of bipolar disorder and a 28.4% risk of unipolar disorder among relatives of unipolar probands. Although the unipolar diagnosis did not require recurrent episodes, the relatives' risk of bipolar disorder does not suggest a familial link between the two disorders. In contrast, the 28.4% risk of unipolar disorder provides strong evidence for familial transmission.

Data obtained from family studies of mood disorder indicate that bipolar disorder is familial. The reported risks of bipolar disorder among relatives of bipolar probands are consistently greater than the risk to the general population, to relatives of normal controls, and to relatives of unipolar probands. The lower risk of bipolar disorder among relatives of unipolar probands suggests that the two disorders do not have identical familial substrates. The reported risk of unipolar disorder in the population is highly variable. For the uncontrolled studies, it is difficult to state whether relatives of unipolar probands are at increased risk of unipolar disorder. However, the four double-blind, controlled studies consistently found higher rates of unipolar disorder among relatives of unipolar probands in comparison with controls. These provide strong evidence favoring the hypothesis that major depression is familial. These results indicate that a unipolar disorder is 1.7 to 9.7 times more likely to be found among relatives of bipolar probands than among relatives of control probands. Thus all the controlled studies found an excess of unipolar disorder in bipolar proband families. The results of examining bipolar disorder in unipolar proband families are less conclusive.

RELATIVE CONTRIBUTIONS OF GENETIC AND ENVIRONMENTAL FACTORS

After the family study method has been used to establish that a disorder is familial, the next question is: "What are the relative contributions of genetic and environmental factors to disease etiology?" To answer this question, it is necessary to go beyond family studies to twin and adoption studies. The major drawback to using these designs is that they are difficult to implement, chiefly because of the difficulty in finding and collecting appropriate twin and adoption samples. Fortunately, some countries, like Denmark, have extensive adoption and twin registries in addition to psychiatric registries. Linkage of the psychiatric registries with the twin and adoption registries has created unique opportunities for genetic epidemiologic investigations of mood disorders.

Twin Studies

The occurrence of twins provides the perfect clinical opportunity to look at the factors involved in human genetics. Identical or monozygotic (MZ) twins have 100% of their genes in common, while fraternal or dizygotic (DZ) twins have only 50% of their genes in common. Although the two types of twins are significantly different in terms of their genetic makeup, there is an assumption that both MZ and DZ twins share a relatively common environment. The genetic similarity between DZ twins is the same as that between siblings. Since DZ twins are not genetic copies of each other, differences within a twin pair can be due to environmental or genetic factors. However, since MZ twins are genetic copies of each other, environmental influences must be responsible for differences between them. Thus, studies of twins are very informative in comparing the relative contributions of genetic and environmental factors of the etiology of psychiatric disorders.

A twin pair is "concordant" if both twins have a disorder; otherwise, they are "discordant." Thus, concordance rates are often used to summarize twin studies of psychiatric disorders. If we assume that genetic factors are important and that the effects of a common environment are the same for both types of twins, we should expect a higher concordance rate for a disorder in MZ twins as compared with DZ twins. Twin research uses two methods to calculate concordance rates, depending on the method of ascertainment of the twin sample. We compute the "pairwise" concordance rate as the number of twin pairs in which both twins are affected by a disorder. It is the number of twin pairs concordant for the illness divided by the number of concordant pairs plus the number of pairs discordant for the illness. This method of computing is appropriate only when the mode of sampling is single selection—that is, the probability of sampling an ill individual is so low that two ill cotwins are never independently ascertained as probands. However, when this condition does not hold, the "probandwise" concordance rate is the appropriate method of reporting the data. We compute probandwise concordance as the proportion of proband twins that have an ill cotwin. Thus, it is the number of concordant pairs plus the number of concordant pairs in which both the twins are probands divided by the number of concordant pairs plus the number of discordant pairs plus the number of concordant pairs in which both twins are probands.

In addition to concordance rates, we can estimate the heritability of a disorder from twin data. Heritability is a measure of the degree to which genetic factors influence the phenotypic variability of a disorder. Phenotypic variability (V_p) comprises two sources of variance: genetic variability (V_g) and environmental variability (V_e). Partitioning the phenotypic variability in this way assumes that genetic and environmental factors are statistically independent (i.e., $V_p = V_g + V_e$). Heritability in the broad sense (h^2) is the ratio of genetic and phenotypic variances (i.e., $h^2 = V_g/V_p$). Thus, a heritability of zero indicates that there is no genetic variability in the sample under consideration. That does not mean, however, that the etiology of the phenotype can be explained solely by environmental influence. Similarly, a heritability of zero indicates that environmental factors are not relevant to disease etiology or that such factors have no variability in the sample under consideration.

The largest and most methodologically sophisticated twin study to date was performed in Denmark by Bertelsen, Harvald, and Hauge (1977), who identified twins through the Danish Psychiatric Twin Register. The authors stated that their diagnostic criteria "were made quite wide in accordance with the concept of Kraepelin." Probands and their partners had to have been admitted to a hospital because of a disorder with "predominating mood disturbances of universal character, supported by the presence of disturbances of psychomotor and mental activity, characteristic sleep disturbances and diurnal variations, and, furthermore, by a periodic course illness and a tendency to recovery without defect" (Bertelsen, 1985). For 53 of 133 pairs, they assessed zygosity from blood types, tissue types, serum protein variants, and isoenzymes. For the remaining pairs, they assessed zygosity with questions regarding similarity and cases of mistaken identity. The Danish twin study provided exact probandwise concordance rates. The investigators found a probandwise concordance rate for bipolar disorder of 0.67 in MZ twins, which is more than three times greater than for DZ twins with a rate of 0.20. From these data, they calculated the heritability of mood disorder to be 0.59. The details of methods for calculating heritability are beyond the scope of this chapter. However, excellent references for heritability calculation methods and the issues involved in their interpretation and use may be found in Holzinger (1929); Smith (1974); and Reich, James, and Morris (1972).

Figure 1–1 contains results from six different twin studies of broadly defined mood disorders or manic-depressive disorder, which did not distinguish between unipolar and bipolar subforms (Tsuang & Faraone, 1990). This figure illustrates the uniqueness of the twin study design, which is able to separate different components of variance of the disorder. The first part of the bar, with the cross-hatching, indicates in each study what percentage of the variance (V) of the disorder may be attributed to genetic factors (G); the black part of the bar indicates what percentage of the disorder may be attributed to common or shared environmental factors (V_c/V), and the white part

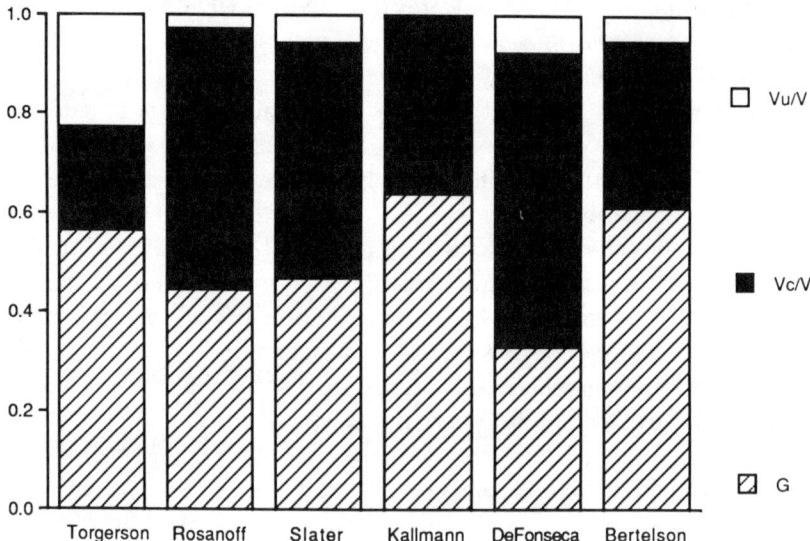

Figure 1–1. Results from six twin studies of mood disorders indicating the relative contributions of genetic (G), common environmental (V_c/V), and unique environmental (V_u/V) factors (from Tsuang & Faraone, 1990).

of the bar indicates the proportion of variance that is accounted for by unique environment factors or events experienced by one twin but not the other (V_u/V). This pattern of results indicates that perhaps 60% of the variance in mood disorders is due to genetic factors, while 30% to 40% of the variance may be attributable to common environmental factors. Unique environmental effects accounted for less than 10% of the variance across these six studies. This is a relatively simple analysis of twin data. However, twin methodology can become quite sophisticated mathematically, and data analyses that include parents and siblings of twins can lead to stronger inferences.

Overall, twin studies of major mood disorders find higher concordance rates for MZ for than DZ twins. The only exception to this is the study of Pollin, Allen, Hoffer, Stabenau, and Hrubec (1969), which used a questionable method of obtaining psychiatric diagnoses. Twin studies are consistent with family studies in suggesting that genetic factors play a substantial role in the mood disorders. However, the finding of MZ concordance rates lower than 100% underscores the importance of environmental factors, including sources of experimental error (e.g., psychiatric, diagnostic, and zygosity misclassification). Twin studies also suggest that common environmental factors account for a sizable component of the etiology. Assortative mating leads to an overestimate of the effects of common environment and an underestimate of heritability. Assortative mating refers to an increased tendency of patients with mood disorders to choose spouses who also have a mood disorder.

Twin studies of minor mood disorders and depressive personality characteristics suggest that such traits have less of a genetic component than do major mood disorders. The studies of Slater and Shields (1969) and of Torgersen (1985) are strikingly consistent in finding a substantial genetic component for anxiety neurosis, but not for depressive neurosis. Twin studies of depressive personality traits have not yet produced consistent results. Two of the three depressive personality studies examining gender as a variable found heritability to be greater for females than for males. This agrees with the findings from Bertelsen and coworkers (1977) unipolar twin sample. However, Clifford, Hopper, Fulker, and Murray (1984) suggest that heritability estimates are inflated due to the effects of shared environment between male and female pairs. Yet this is at variance with the results of Jardine, Martin, and Henderson (1984), who found that familial environmental factors were not important even though the heritability for females was significantly, but not markedly, greater than that for males. We cannot draw firm conclusions about the etiology of gender effects in mood disorders from these mixed sets of results.

Adoption Studies

Adoption studies provide one of the few ways of isolating genetic and environmental contributions to the familial transmission of a disorder. The adoption study design can indicate whether biological or adoptive relationships primarily account for the transmission of disorders, because the possibility of postnatal environmental interaction between the adopted child and the child's biological relatives is removed. This is true because children adopted at an early age have a primarily genetic relationship with their biological parents and an environmental relationship with their adoptive parents. There is some possibility that the biological relatives had some early environmental influence; one example is poor prenatal and perinatal care, which can cause environmental insults to the newborn. Such factors confound the genetic parent–child relationship. However, despite the potential for confounding and the difficulty of ascertaining an appropriate sample, the thoughtful implementation of an adoption study constitutes a valuable tool for teasing apart genetic and environmental contributions.

There are three major designs for adoption studies: the adoptee-as-proband design, the parent-as-proband design, and the cross-fostering design. The adoptee-as-proband design uses ill and well probands. A genetic component is indicated if the biological relatives of ill adoptees are shown to have a greater propensity for illness than the adoptive relatives of ill adoptees. The parent-as-proband design compares the incidence of illness in adopted children of ill and well individuals. A genetic component is indicated if the risk of illness among adopted children of ill individuals is greater than the risk to adopted children of well individuals. Last, the cross-fostering design compares a group of probands who have ill biological parents but are raised by well adoptive parents with a group of probands who have well biological parents but are raised by ill adoptive parents. This design, in particular, allows one directly to compare environmental and biological transmission in an adoptee sample.

When examining adoption studies, one must remember that adoptees and their families are not representative of the general population. They are the exception rather than the rule in terms of psychiatric morbidity. For example, children who have a diagnosis of attention-deficit disorder according to the third edition of the *Diagnostic and Statistical Manual of Mental Disorders* (DSM-III) are eight times more likely to have been adopted than children with no psychiatric disorders (Deutsch et al., 1982). The causes of increased psychiatric illness among adoptees and their relatives are unknown. Both genetic and environmental factors may play a role. It is very likely that parents who have a mental disorder are more inclined to put their children up for adoption than are parents who have no mental disorder. It also may be the case that the stress of being an adoptee may contribute to the prevalence of mental disorders. Because of these factors, it is especially important to include an adoptee control group in the methodological design of adoption studies.

The first reported adoption study of mood disorders was conducted by Mendlewicz and Rainer (1977) in Belgium. They used the adoptee-as-proband design with the addition of two control groups—the parents of the nonadoptees with mood disorder and the parents of poliomyelitis patients. The researchers chose this latter group to control for the effect on parents of raising a disabled child. The incidence of psychiatric illness was found to be greater among the biological than among the adoptive parents of bipolar adoptees. The results for the biological parents of bipolar nonadoptees indicate an increased risk of mood disorders in these relatives. The results for adoptive parents of bipolar adoptees indicate that adoptive relationships do not mediate the familial risk for developing mood disorders. Additionally, there is no indication that the stress of raising a child with a disabling disease such as poliomyelitis significantly increases the risk of having a mental disorder. Overall, the results implicate genetic factors in the familial transmission of mood disorders.

Cadoret (1978) used a parent-as-proband design to compare eight adoptees whose biological mothers had mood disorders with 118 adoptees whose biological mothers did not have mood disorders. There were no cases of bipolar disorder among the adoptees. However, the rate of unipolar disorder was much higher among adoptees with ill biological mothers (38%) as compared with those having well biological mothers (9%). Because of the small sample size, the difference was not statistically significant, and thus results are difficult to interpret. In another study, Cadoret, O'Gorman, Heywood, and Troughton (1985) interviewed 443 adoptees and their adoptive parents and assessed biological relatives based on adoption agency, hospital, or court records. Adoptees with a biological family history of mood disorder were more likely to have had an episode of illness as compared with adoptees with no such family history. However, the difference was not statistically significant. In contrast, some environmental characteristics of the adoptive family were predictive of adoptee depression, including alcohol abuse by the adoptive parents, other psychiatric illness in the adoptive parents, and death of an adoptive parent.

Wender and colleagues (1986) used the adoptee-as-proband design for their study, which was conducted in Denmark. The investigators identified 71 adult adoptees with mood disorders and 75 control adoptees with no record of psychiatric illness. They matched the ill and control adoptees on sex, age, time spent with biological mother, age at transfer to adoptive home, and socioeconomic class of the adopting parents. Owing to the precise and extensive network of the Danish registry system, they were able to identify 387 biological relatives of ill adoptees, 344 biological relatives of control adoptees, 180 adoptive relatives of ill adoptees, and 169 adoptive relatives of control adoptees. Among relatives of ill adoptees, the risk to biological relatives was greater than the risk to adoptive relatives. Notably, the biological relatives of ill adoptees were six times more likely than the adoptive relatives to have completed suicide, and had three times the rate of unipolar disorder and alcoholism.

In summary, adoption studies of the major mood disorders have yielded inconsistent results. Although two studies strongly support the genetic hypothesis (Mendlewicz & Rainer, 1977; Wender et al., 1986), more adoption studies are needed to strengthen the assertion that genetic factors play a substantial role in the etiology of mood disorders. It would be of particular interest to conduct a cross-fostering study, because the design has not yet been used to examine the genetics of mood disorders.

DETERMINING THE MODE OF GENETIC TRANSMISSION

Traditionally, the method of establishing the mode of genetic transmission for a disorder has been to apply sophisticated mathematical models to family data in an attempt to describe the distribution of illness in families. Genetic epidemiologists developed this type of mathematical modeling, known as segregation analysis, to determine whether the distribution of illness in families was consistent with a single gene, many genes (polygenic), many genes along with the environment (multifactorial polygenic), or environmental transmission alone. Recently, it has become feasible to use linkage analysis to find genes that predispose to familial diseases (discussed elsewhere in this volume).

There are two statistical procedures used to model genetic transmission, prevalence analysis and pedigree segregation analysis. The major difference between the two approaches involves the form in which the family data enter the analysis. Prevalence analyses reduce the data to a matrix that specifies the prevalence of the disorder in relatives of ill and control probands (Reich et al., 1972; Reich, James, & Morris, 1979). This form of analysis loses important information about the familial pattern of illness in a given sample because it does not treat probands with multiple ill relatives differently from those with only one relative. The method of pedigree segregation analysis (Elston, 1981) uses all such information available in the pedigree to test genetic hypotheses. Pedigree segregation analysis also has greater statistical power than does prevalence analysis (Kidd, 1981). A genetic model has two major aspects: a description of how the disorder is transmitted and a procedure for determining whether the predictions made by the model are adequate descriptions of the observed familial patterns of the disorder.

Single major locus (SML) models propose that a pair of alleles is responsible for the transmission of a disorder. If b represents the pathogenic or predisposing allele and B represents the normal allele at the same locus, then there are three possible genotypes at the single major locus: BB, Bb, and bb. According to the classic Mendelian rules of inheritance, if the gene is recessive, then all individuals with the bb genotype will have the disorder and the other two genotypes will be unaffected. If the gene is dominant, the affected genotypes include both bb and Bb. From family, twin, and adoption data, we know that the major mood disorders do not follow a simple Mendelian mode of inheritance. In pedigree segregation analysis, the statistical SML model may be modified by incorporating a number of additional parameters to account for non-Mendelian distributions of disorders within families. For instance, we can modify the penetrance, that is, the probability that an individual with the vulnerable genotype will manifest the disorder. In this manner, we can model environmental factors that influence the expression of the disorder. Also, we can add a parameter to account for disorders that exhibit a variable age of onset.

The issue of polygenic inheritance is a potential problem for both segregation analysis and linkage analysis. For example, if a disorder is caused by 10 genes, each of these genes will be difficult to find unless one or two of them have a major effect. For polygenic disorders, currently available segregation and linkage methods may not be helpful. There are two classes of polygenic models. Limited loci polygenic (LLP) models propose that a relatively limited number of genes are responsible for a disorder. The extreme case of an LLP model is the multifactorial polygenic (MFP) model. These models propose that a large, unspecified number of genes and environmental factors are responsible. Because there are many possible two-locus models that can describe dichotomous traits, LLP models are difficult to test (Elston & Namboodiri, 1977). Even when a plausible argument can be made for excluding many of these possibilities because they either do not fit hypotheses about the disorder or are biologically meaningless, the number of models that remain to be tested is overwhelming.

The MFP model is more manageable despite the large number of components involved. Although the model posits that many genes and environmental factors contribute to disease causation, they are not enumerated and none is individually necessary or sufficient. According to the model, a hypothetical construct called liability, made up of numerous genetic and environmental components, is normally distributed. Individuals above a certain threshold on the liability scale manifest the disorder. To represent varying degrees of severity, we place more than one threshold along the liability continuum, see Figure 1–2. Individuals on the right of the right-hand threshold will

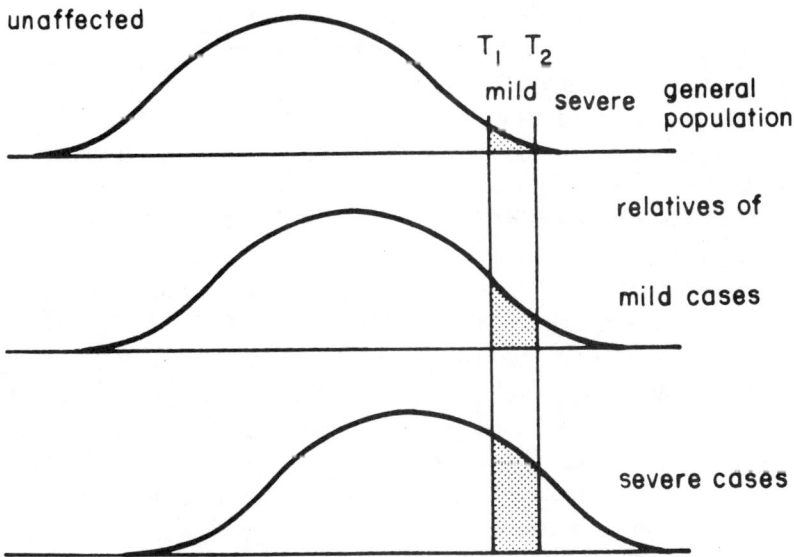

Figure 1–2. Overview of multiple threshold multifactorial model of genetic transmission. From top to bottom, the three curves indicate the distributions of genetic liability in the general population, among relatives of mild cases of illness, and among relatives of severe cases of illness (see text for further explanation).

develop the severe form of the disorder; in some contexts, this would be bipolar disorder. Those whose liability falls between the two thresholds would have a less severe form, such as unipolar major depression. Those to the left of the left-hand threshold would have a minor form (e.g., mild depression) or be unaffected.

The multiple-threshold MFP model predicts that an individual's risk for the disorder increases as a function of the severity of the illness in his or her relatives, and that an individual with many affected relatives carries a higher risk than someone with few affected relatives. This occurs when those individuals with more genes have more severe forms of the illness. The pedigree segregation analysis formulation of the MFP model is unable to separate and evaluate the relative contributions of genetic and environmental effects. In contrast, path-analytic MFP models can disentangle these factors. These models use the technique of path analysis to partition the observed illness correlations between family members into several components. For instance, the correlations between members of a family might be partitioned into five components: (1) the effect of transmissible environment on phenotype (cultural heritability); (2) the effect of genotype on phenotype (the genetic heritability); (3) the effect on phenotype of environmental factors unique to twins; (4) the effect of transmissible parental environment on the transmissible environment of a child raised by the parent; and (5) the correlation between the transmissible environments of each parent (i.e., nonrandom mating). The mixed model posits that both MFP and SML components may be involved in disease etiology. Statistical analysis of the mixed model can determine whether either component alone can provide an adequate fit to the data or if the null hypothesis of no SML effect and no MFP effect fits best.

Unfortunately, mathematical analyses of mood disorder pedigrees have not been able to support consistently a mode of genetic transmission for either unipolar or bipolar mood disorders. Indeed, as two reviews indicate, there is no strong support for either single-gene or polygenic transmission, even when such factors as gender and polarity are taken into account in the analyses (Tsuang & Faraone, 1990; Faraone, Kremen, & Tsuang, 1990). This suggests that mathematical genetic modeling studies have reached a limit in their utility for understanding the transmission of major mood disorders. It may be that better definitions of genetic variants of mood disorder are needed before such studies are worthwhile. While methodological improvements in terms of the collection of family data have strengthened this approach, they do not directly address what is perhaps the most important issue, the problem of determining the appropriate specification of the phenotype.

Despite advances in psychiatric nosology, there is still much work to be done in the classification of psychiatric disorders into genetically homogeneous subgroups. Perhaps when we are able to combine traditional diagnostic techniques with the assessment of biological markers, phenotype specification will approach the standards of reliability and validity necessary for statistical modeling techniques to be useful in psychiatry.

The mode of inheritance of mood disorders has substantial implications for etiological research and clinical practice. Conclusive evidence implicating a single major locus would facilitate pathophysiological research. Indeed, the discovery of a DNA mutation that causes illness could lead to a direct biochemical pathway from genotype to phenotype.

SUMMARY AND CONCLUSIONS

The risk of mood disorders increases with the proportion of genes shared with a mood-disordered patient. The risk to relatives is higher than the risk to the general population. It is also higher than the risk to relatives of well individuals as determined by double-blind, case-controlled studies. Thus, family data unequivocally indicate that mood disorders are familial, that is, they run in families.

The concordance rate for mood disorder among monozygotic twins is approximately three times the rate observed among dizygotic twins. This strongly suggests that genes play a crucial role in the familial transmission of these disorders. The MZ twin concordance rate is approximately 0.70 for bipolar disorder and 0.50 for unipolar disorder. Since concordance is not perfect, nonfamilial environmental factors must play a role in the etiology of mood disorders. These factors appear to be less prominent for bipolar than for unipolar disorder. The conclusions from the twin studies agree with two methodologically strong adoption studies indicating that biological relationships are better predictors of the risk of mood disorders than are adoptive relationships—that is, both types of study suggest that the familial transmission of these disorders has a primarily genetic source. The environmental factors that cause illness are likely to be nonfamilial. However, since the adoption study literature contains some conflicting reports, we need more adoption studies to provide convergent support for these assertions.

The genetic relationship between unipolar and bipolar disorders is poorly understood. Further research into this area must distinguish recurrent unipolar cases that are not likely to have a subsequent manic episode from nonrecurrent cases that may be bipolar. It is probably true that cases of unipolar disorder within families that manifest bipolar disorder are genetic variants of bipolar disorder. The clearest and most consistent difference between the two forms of mood disorder is that relatives of bipolar probands are at a greater risk for both unipolar and bipolar disorders than are relatives of unipolar probands. Evidence from both family and twin studies supports this conclusion. Thus, it is likely that bipolar disorder has a greater familial component than does unipolar disorder; unipolar appears to be more greatly affected by nonfamilial, environmental factors.

Despite strong evidence for a genetic component to mood disorders, mathematical modeling studies do not consistently support a specific mode of genetic transmission. Also, as indicated elsewhere in this volume, linkage studies have led to equivocal results. Since mathematical modeling and linkage analyses have tested relatively simple models of genetic transmission, it may be that more complex models are needed to describe the transmission of mood disorders or that advances in nosology are needed to define genetic variants of these disorders.

REFERENCES

Andreasen, N. C., Rice, J., Endicott, J., Coryell, W., Grove, W. M., & Reich, T. (1987). Familial rates of affective disorder: A report from the National Institute of Mental Health Collaborative Study. *Archives of General Psychiatry, 44,* 461–469.

Bertelsen, A. (1985). A Danish twin study of manic-depressive disorders. In T. Sakai & T. Tsubsi (Eds.), *Genetic aspects of human behavior* (pp. 97–102). New York: Igaku-Shoin.

Bertelsen, A., Harvald, B., & Hauge, M. (1977). A Danish twin study of manic-depressive disorders. *British Journal of Psychiatry, 130,* 330–351.

Cadoret, R. J. (1978). Evidence for genetic inheritance of primary affective disorder in adoptees. *American Journal of Psychiatry, 135,* 463–466.

Cadoret, R. J., O'Gorman, T. W., Heywood, E., & Troughton, E. (1985). Genetic and environmental factors in major depression. *Journal of Affective Disorders, 9,* 155–164.

Clifford, C. A., Hopper, J. L., Fulker, D. W., & Murray, R. M. (1984). A genetic and environmental analysis of a twin family study of alcohol use, anxiety and depression. *Genetic Epidemiology, 1,* 63–79.

Deutsch, C. K., Swanson, J. M., Bruell, J. H., Cantwell, D. P., Weinberg, F., & Baren, M. (1982). Short communication: Overrepresentation of adoptees in children with attention deficit disorder. *Behavior Genetics, 12,* 231–238.

Egeland, J. A., & Hostetter, A. M. (1983). Amish study: I. Affective disorders among the Amish. *American Journal of Psychiatry, 140,* 56–61.

Elston, R. C. (1981). Segregation analysis. In H. Harris & K. Hirschorn (Eds.), *Advances in human genetics* (pp. 63–120). New York: Plenum.

Elston, R. C., & Namboodiri, K. K. (1977). Family studies of schizophrenia. *Bulletin of the International Statistics Institute, 47,* 683–697.

Endicott, J., Nee, J., Andreasen, N., Clayton, P., Keller, M., & Coryell, W. (1985). Bipolar II: Combine or separate? *Journal of Affective Disorders, 8,* 17–28.

Essen-Moller, E., & Hagnell, O. (1961). The frequency and risk of depression within a rural population group in Scandinavia. *Acta Psychiatrica Scandinavica, Suppl., 162,* 28–32.

Faraone, S. V., Kremen, W. S., & Tsuang, M. T. (1990). Genetic transmission of major affective disorders: Quantitative models and linkage analyses. *Psychological Bulletin, 108,* 109–127.

Fremming, G. H. (1951). *The expectation of mental infirmity in a sample of the Danish population.* London: Cassell.

Gershon, E. S., Baron, M., & Leckman, J. F. (1975). Genetic models of the transmission of affective disorders. *Journal of Psychiatric Research, 12,* 301–317.

Gershon, E. S., Hamovit, J., Guroff, J. J., Dibble, E., Leckman, J. F., Sceery, W., Targum, S. D., Nurnberger, J. I., Jr., Goldin, L. R., & Bunney, W. E., Jr. (1982). A family study of schizoaffective bipolar I, bipolar II, unipolar and normal control probands. *Archives of General Psychiatry, 39,* 1157–1167.

Gershon, E. S., Hamovit, J. H., Guroff, J. J., & Nurnberger, J. I., Jr. (1987). Birth-cohort changes in manic and depressive disorders in relatives of bipolar and schizoaffective patients. *Archives of General Psychiatry, 44,* 314–319.

Hagnell, O., Lanke, J., Rorsman, B., & Ojesio, L. (1982). Are we entering an age of melancholy? Depressive illness in a prospective epidemiological study over 25 years: Lundby study. *Psychological Medicine, 12,* 122–129.

Helgason, T. (1961). Frequency of depressive states within geographically delimited population groups: The frequency of depressive states in Iceland as compared with the other Scandinavian countries. *Acta Psychiatrica Scandinavica, Suppl., 162,* 81–90.

Helgason, T. (1979). Epidemiological investigations concerning affective disorders. In M. Schou, & E. Stromgren (Eds.), *Origin prevention and treatment of affective disorders.* New York: Academic Press.

Holzinger, K. J. (1929). The relative effect of nature and nurture on twin differences. *Journal of Educational Psychology, 20,* 241–248.

James, N. M., & Chapman, C. J. (1975). A genetic study of bipolar affective disorder. *American Journal of Psychiatry, 126,* 449–456.

Jardine, R., Martin, N. G., & Henderson, A. S. (1984). Genetic covariation between neuroticism and the symptoms of anxiety and depression. *Genetic Epidemiology, 1,* 89–107.

Kidd, K. K. (1981). Genetic models for psychiatric disorders. In E. S. Gershon, S. Mathysee, X. O. Breakefield, & R. D. Ciaranello (Eds.), *Genetic research strategies for psychobiology and psychiatry* (pp. 369–382). New York: Boxwood.

Klerman, G. L. (1976). Age and clinical depression: Today's youth in the twenty-first century. *Journal of Gerontology, 31,* 318–323.

Klerman, G. L., Lavori, P. W., Rice, J., Reich, T., Endicott, J., Andreasen, N. C., Keller, M. B., & Hirschfield, R. M. A. (1985). Birth-cohort trends in rates of major depressive disorder among relatives of patients with affective disorder. *Archives of General Psychiatry, 42,* 689–693.

Lavori, P. W., Klerman, G. L., Keller, M. B., Reich, T., Rice, J., & Endicott, J. (1986). Age-period-cohort analysis of secular trends in onset of major depression: Findings in siblings of patients with major affective disorder. *Journal of Psychiatric Research, 21,* 23–35.

Mendlewicz, J., & Rainer, J. D. (1977). Adoption study supporting genetic transmission in manic-depressive illness. *Nature, 268,* 327–329.

Morton, N. E. (1982). Outline of genetic epidemiology. Basel: Karger.

Parsons, P. L. (1965). Mental health of Swansea's old folk. *British Journal of Preventative Social Medicine, 19,* 43–47.

Perris, C. (1966). A study of bipolar (manic-depressive) and unipolar recurrent depressive psychoses. *Acta Psychiatrica Scandinavica, 42* (suppl. 194), 1–188.

Pollin, W., Allen, M. G., Hoffer, A., Stabenau, J. R., & Hrubec, Z. (1969). Psychopathology in 15,909 pairs of veteran twins: Evidence for a genetic factor in the pathogenesis of schizophrenia and its relative absence in psychoneurosis. *American Journal of Psychiatry, 126,* 597–610.

Reich, T., James, J. W., & Morris, C. (1972). The use of multiple thresholds in determining the mode of transmission of semi-continuous traits. *Annals of Human Genetics, 36,* 163–184.

Reich, T., James, J. W., & Morris, C. (1979). The use of multiple thresholds in determining the mode of transmission of semi-continuous traits. *Annals of Human Genetics, 42,* 371–389.

Rice, J., Reich, T., Andreasen, N. C., Endicott, J., Van Eerdewegh, M., Fishman, R., Hirschfeld, R. M. A., & Klerman, G. L. (1987). The familial transmission of bipolar illness. *Archives of General Psychiatry, 44,* 441–447.

Robins, L. N., Heltzer, J. E., Weissman, M. M., Orvaschel, H., Gruenberg, E., Burke, J. D., Ir, & Regier, D. A. (1984). Lifetime prevalence of specific psychiatric disorders in three sites. *Archives of General Psychiatry, 41,* 949–958.

Slater, E., & Shields, J. (1969). Genetic aspects of anxiety. In M. Lader (Ed.), Studies of anxiety. *British Journal of Psychiatry, Spec. Pub. No. 3,* 62–71.

Smeraldi, E., Negri, F., & Melica, A. M. (1977). A genetic study of affective disorders. *Acta Psychiatrica Scandinavica, 56,* 382–399.

Smith, C. (1974). Concordance in twins: Methods and interpretation. *American Journal of Human Genetics, 26,* 454–466.

Srole, L., & Fischer, A. (1980). The midtown Manhattan longitudinal study vs. the mental paradise lost doctrine. *Archives of General Psychiatry, 37,* 209–221.

Torgersen, S. (1985). Hereditary differentiation of anxiety and neuroses. *British Journal of Psychiatry, 146,* 530–534.

Trzebiatowska-Trzeciak, O. (1977). Genetic analysis of unipolar and bipolar endogenous affective psychoses. *British Journal of Psychiatry, 131,* 478–485.

Tsuang, M. T., & Faraone, S. V. (1990). *The genetics of mood disorders.* Baltimore, MD: Johns Hopkins Press.

Tsuang, M. T., Winokur, G., & Crowe, R. R. (1980). Morbidity risks of schizophrenia and affective disorders among first-degree relatives of patients with schizophrenia, mania, depression, and surgical conditions. *British Journal of Psychiatry, 137,* 497–504.

Weissman, M. M., Gershon, E. S., Kidd, K. K., Prusoff, B. A., Leckman, J. F., Dibble, E., Hamovit, J., Thompson, W. D., Pauls, D. L., & Guroff, J. J. (1984). Psychiatric disorders in the relatives of probands with affective disorders: The Yale-NIMH collaborative study. *Archives of General Psychiatry, 41,* 13–21.

Weissman, M. M., & Myers, J. K. (1978). Affective disorders in a U.S. urban community: The use of research diagnostic criteria in an epidemiological survey. *Archives of General Psychiatry, 35,* 1304–1311.

Wender, P. H., Kety, S. S., Rosenthal, D., Schulsinger, F., Ortmann, J., & Lunde, I. (1986). Psychiatric disorders in the biological and adoptive families and adopted individuals with affective disorders. *Archives of General Psychiatry, 43,* 923–929.

2

Diagnostic Issues in Pedigree Assessment

JEAN ENDICOTT AND MIRON BARON

There are no laboratory tests to aid in the diagnosis of the conditions now considered best classified among the affective, or mood, disorders. Diagnostic evaluation depends on an assessment of clinical phenomenology and the course of illness. The lack of laboratory tests is coupled with the problem of phenotypic uncertainty regarding which conditions should be considered part of the spectrum of disorders to be included as "affected" in genetic linkage studies of affective disorders.

In addition, given the high rates of affective disorder in the community and the results of family studies, as well as studies on the course of illness and the different responses to treatments, there is a widely held assumption that more than one "type" of affective disorder exists and that there may be different genetic forms even among patients who have the most similar phenotypes. As will be noted, investigators who attempt to study even the most classic forms of bipolar disorder with mania (referred to hereafter as bipolar I disorder) are confronted with a host of problems related to possible heterogeneity.

This chapter focuses on a number of issues related to diagnostic assessment, using the study of bipolar I disorder as the prototypic condition to illustrate the decisions that must be made by investigators who are conducting genetic linkage studies. These include those issues related to the initial selection of the families, those regarding which conditions will be considered "affected" for the analyses, and those determining how to collect and record the diagnostic information. No attempt will be made to discuss issues related to the advantages and disadvantages or analytic implications of different (1) sampling techniques or (2) means of taking into account the "uncertain" cases. However, any investigator considering genetic linkage studies should be aware of these, and other issues as well, since they have major design and operational implications (Merikangas, Spenec, & Kupfer, 1989).

DIAGNOSTIC CRITERIA FOR INITIAL SELECTION OF FAMILIES

There is no "golden rule" for the initial selection of families to be studied. However, most investigators wish to have some evidence that the family is sufficiently "loaded" with the condition of interest to be potentially informative in the linkage analyses. Usually they want to select families with at least three members who have the "core" disorder, ideally involving more than one generation. Other criteria with regard to family size, number of potential sib-pairs, need for bilineal descent, and so on, are more variable.

Most linkage studies of affective disorders conducted to date have focused on bipolar I disorder as the primary condition of interest in the initial selection of the families to be included. Even here, where there is little disagreement regarding the basic phenomenologic criteria of a manic syndrome, there is variation in the form, course, and severity of clinical manifestations and questions regarding the best forms to include as the initial selection criteria. For example, should the proband and the two or three other key relatives required for selection of the family all have had an early onset of bipolar I disorder? Should there be evidence that the manic syndrome developed in the absence of any "provocative" stimulus, such as medication, drug abuse, or some premorbid medical condition? Should there be evidence that the disorder is recurrent, that is, is not limited to a single episode?

These questions, and others to be noted below, are of importance, even in the initial selection of the families for study, because of the recognition that there is some likelihood that there might be phenocopies of even the more restrictive definitions of the core condition under study. Such phenocopies of the condition—that is, the presence of the clinical syndrome but not of the genetic form of the disorder under study—could have a particularly deleterious effect on the efforts to establish linkage if they were introduced during the initial selection of the families to be studied.

In contrast to a number of the other conditions often included in the spectrum of affective disorders, there is little disagreement regarding the clinical phenomena of the inclusion criteria for a manic syndrome. The agreement as to what constitutes a manic syndrome is generally high across different diagnostic systems and among raters. However, there is some disagreement with regard to the weight given various clinical features, particularly in the initial selection of the families. Should elation, or at least expansiveness, be required as a prominent symptom or it is sufficient to be irritable and angry? Should there be evidence of less need for sleep or is increased activity sufficient? How long should the syndrome last in the absence of treatment or with treatment?

There is more disagreement regarding the exclusion criteria. Should subjects who also meet one or more sets of criteria for schizoaffective disorder be excluded in the initial selection of the families? If a decision is made to include all or some of those who meet the phenomenological criteria for schizoaffective disorder one must consider the inclusion or exclusion of different subtypes based on the type of affective syndrome (depression only or mania and depression) and course of illness, particularly the relative prominence of the affective and schizophrenic-like symptoms (e.g., subtypes of mainly affective or mainly schizophrenic).

These kinds of decisions should be made in advance by the investigator. They should be based on an understanding of the evidence of the likely heritability of the condition when the criteria selected for inclusion and exclusion are used.

SELECTION OF DISORDERS TO BE INCLUDED IN THE SPECTRUM AS AFFECTED

Very few families would be informative for genetic linkage studies if the investigator were to restrict the study to cases that only met the inclusion criteria for the core condition initially used to select the families for study. It is usually necessary to count as affected a number of conditions that are assumed to be within the bipolar spectrum, that is, different manifestations of the same condition as the core disorder. In the absence of laboratory tests or other markers of the disorder, investigators must weigh other evidence in deciding which conditions to include. Even after deciding which conditions are to be included within the spectrum, the investigator must further decide whether to include them in the more narrow or the broader diagnostic hierarchies used in successive analyses of the data derived from the pedigree study.

The classic criterion for inclusion of a disorder in a spectrum of disorders has been evidence of differential familial aggregation—that is, the condition appears with higher frequency in families with the core condition of interest than in the families of an appropriate control group. The strongest evidence of familial aggregation is derived from twin studies, contrasting the rates for monozygotic with those of same sex dizygotic twins or siblings. Other high-risk studies, such as those of children of affected parents, offer supportive evidence for the inclusion or exclusion of candidate disorders. In evaluating the results of these studies, the investigator must be aware of the possible effects of comorbid conditions in the index subjects, as well as the possibility of assortative mating in the parents of the subjects. The greater the degree to which there is evidence from studies that support the inclusion of a disorder within the spectrum, the more confident the investigator may be that the condition is indeed related to (or is a form of) the core condition. For example, several studies have supported the inclusion of the bipolar form or schizoaffective disorder in the spectrum with bipolar I disorder (Gershon et al., 1982; Endicott et al., 1985; Rice et al., 1987).

Another criterion for inclusion in the spectrum is evidence that one condition is likely to be an early manifestation of the core condition or one of the other disorders that are higher in the hierarchy. The evidence for such an association usually comes from prospective studies, with repeated careful diagnostic evaluations performed by clinicians who are unaware of the diagnoses made previously. For example, some subjects with early manifestations of hypomania are likely later to become manic.

The investigator should be aware that most of the other candidate disorders for inclusion in the spectrum are more common than the core condition, more diagnostically problematic, and more likely to include phenocopies or false positives (even if some forms of these disorders are indeed part of the spectrum).

OTHER TYPES OF MAJOR AFFECTIVE DISORDER

In considering the conditions most likely to be among those genetically related to bipolar I disorder, those first considered include the bipolar forms of schizoaffective disorder (as mentioned above), bipolar disorder with hypomania, and unipolar depressive disorder.

Bipolar Schizoaffective Disorder

Many investigators include the bipolar forms of schizoaffective disorder as part of the core condition, having decided on clinical grounds that they are just a more severe form of psychotic manic disorder. Others limit the inclusion to those instances in which the disorder appears to have recurrences and remissions without evidence of schizophrenic-like symptoms or functioning during periods when the full affective syndrome (either manic or depressive) is absent. As noted above, there is also some research evidence to support the inclusion of some cases of bipolar schizoaffective disorder as affected within highly loaded bipolar pedigrees.

Bipolar Disorder with Hypomania

It has long been recognized that many patients who experience periods of major depressive syndrome also have periods of hypomania in the absence of periods of mania (bipolar II disorder). Patients with bipolar II disorder are frequently found among the first-degree relatives of bipolar I patients. However, recently there have been studies that have suggested that bipolar II disorder may breed true and not simply be a less pronounced or milder manifestation of bipolar I disorder (Endicott et al., 1985; Coryell, Endicott, Reich, Andreasen, & Keller, 1984; Coryell, Endicott, Andreasen, & Keller, 1985; Rice, Reich, Andreason, Coryell, & Endicott, 1984; Rice et al., 1987). There is also evidence from follow-up studies that it is only occasionally an early form of bipolar I disorder (Coryell, Keller, Endicott, & Andreasen, 1989). These studies have led to some disagreement regarding the wisdom of including the condition as affected in the bipolar I linkage studies. However, most investigators consider it a part of the spectrum—particularly if the family has initially been selected on the basis of multiple family members having had a manic syndrome.

There are problems with the test-retest assessments of current or past hypomania that are reflected in lower kappa coefficients of reliability than is the case for bipolar I disorder (Rice et al., 1986). Many investigators take this into account in their placement of bipolar II disorder in the different diagnostic hierarchies, putting it in the broader rather than the narrowest category. They may place bipolar II disorder with major depressive episode(s) in a narrower classification of affected than bipolar II disorder with minor depressive episodes or unipolar hypomanic episodes only.

Unipolar Depressive Disorder

Of the major affective disorders, this is the condition that has the potential to produce the greatest number of false positives in the linkage analyses. Families selected on the basis of one or more cases with a history of manic syndromes will usually have more members with unipolar depressive disorder than with either bipolar I or bipolar II disorder. This is not always the case, but it is rare to find families such as those in the Amish linkage study (Egeland et al., 1991) in which more of the affected showed evidence of mania or hypomania than of unipolar depression alone. The fact that the unipolar form of the disorder is more frequent would not present a problem if there were not also evidence that there are unipolar forms of major affective disorder that seem to have no genetic relationship to bipolar affective disorder.

There have been many efforts to identify clinical features or aspects of the course of the unipolar depressive disorder that might better identify the bipolar-related forms. To date, the two features most widely accepted are those of early onset and recurrence. Some investigators put these forms of Unipolar Depressive Disorder in the narrower categories of affected and the single-episode or late-onset forms in the broader categories for inclusion in later analyses.

Some clinicians and investigators have noted that a large percentage of patients with bipolar I or bipolar II disorders at times manifest reverse vegetative symptoms (Detre et al., 1972). During some depressive periods, they are more likely to have hypersomnia and increased appetite (often with carbohydrate craving). During those periods, they are also more likely to have reactive rather than autonomous and stable depressive mood. Although one might consider using such atypical features to upgrade the classification of some patients with unipolar depressive disorder from a broader to a narrower diagnostic class, apparently none of the investigators working on the genetics of bipolar I disorder have yet done so. Certainly, such atypical clinical features should cue the diagnostician to inquire in even greater detail regarding the possible occurrence prior hypomanic or manic periods.

Recurrent Unipolar Schizoaffective Disorder

Some investigators exclude unipolar schizoaffective disorder from all categories of affected in their studies of families selected for studies of bipolar I disorder. However, given the difficulties of reliably differentiating the psychotic forms of unipolar depressive disorder from those of unipolar schizoaffective disorder, and the results of family and twin studies, most investigators include such cases as affected—although, the recurrent forms are usually placed in a narrower category of affected than the single-episode or more chronic forms of the disorder.

NON-MAJOR AFFECTIVE DISORDERS

There are a number of conditions that might be part of the spectrum of disorders related to bipolar I disorder. For the most part, they are less reliably diagnosed, there is less evidence from the family and twin studies for their inclusion, and the prospective studies on course of illness are less supportive for their inclusion. They include minor depressive disorders, labile personality, and cyclothymia.

Minor Depressive Disorder

Most investigators classify patients with minor depressive disorders as "unaffected," while others place such cases in an "uncertain" category, particularly if the episodes are recurrent. To date, the evidence suggests that, in most instances, minor depressive episodes are unrelated to the likely occurrence of major affective disorders in family members. Furthermore, they are not highly predictive of the subsequent occurrence of episodes of major affective disorder in the subject.

Labile Personality

This unofficial diagnostic category has not been studied extensively. Although many clinicians report an association with bipolar affective disorders (within the subject or the family), most investigators classify individuals with this condition as "unaffected" or "uncertain" in their analyses.

Cyclothymia

Although the clinical features of cyclothymia resemble those of hypomania and minor depressive syndromes, the cyclic nature of the condition and the increased frequency of its occurrence in the families of patients with bipolar I disorder have led to the frequently held assumption that it should be included in the spectrum of bipolar disorders. Unfortunately, the test-retest reliability of this diagnosis is lower than that of major affective disorders. This lower reliability and the less severe nature of the condition have led to its placement in the broad categories of affected but general exclusion from the narrower groupings.

THE NEED FOR NARROW AND BROADER GROUPINGS OF DISORDERS

The incorrect placement of a disorder in the spectrum to be considered "affected" for a particular set of analyses designed to detect evidence of linkage can be quite costly. The cost of misclassification of an individual as unaffected when the appropriate classification should be affected (false negative) is not very high unless (1) the subject is older and well past the usual age of risk, (2) the penetrance estimates used in the analyses are high, or (3) the subject with the disorder is in a key position in the pedigree. All of these circumstances can falsely reduce the evidence for linkage. In contrast, the cost of false positive cases (i.e., those misclassified as affected when the disorder should not be considered part of the spectrum, or when the subject is misdiagnosed as having a spectrum disorder) is much greater since such misclassification can lead to mistaken rejection of genuine linkage. It is because of these consequences and their effects on the linkage analyses that most investigators initially use a limited or narrow group of disorders for their analyses and only later, if evidence suggestive of linkage is found, do they move to a more inclusive (i.e., broader) grouping.

An example of four sets of diagnostic hierarchies for genetic studies of bipolar I disorder, noting which are considered affected and which are uncertain, is shown in Table 2–1. These are the groupings of research diagnostic criteria (RDC) disorders currently being used by the authors and their colleagues (Baron & Endicott, 1990; Baron et al., 1990). While the disorders included in the first set, the narrowest, would be endorsed by most investigators performing linkage studies of bipolar I disorder, the assignment of specific disorders to the successively broader groupings undoubtedly would differ. For example, some investigators might add specific restrictions based on age at onset or recurrence, while others would use different combinations of disorders, particularly in the two middle groupings.

This table also reflects the use of procedures whereby the diagnoses may be made at three levels of certainty: definite, probable, and clinical. (Some investigators use the term possible instead of clinical.) These distinctions are made in recognition of the fact that, given the information available for a particular individual in the pedigree, the certainty with which the diagnostician can make the diagnosis for particular disorders will vary. "Definite" generally means that the certainty of diagnostic fit to the particular set of criteria being employed is quite good and is well documented. The label of "probable" is often used when the subject does not meet the specific criteria for definite but does meet specific criteria for probable, or when the diagnostician is not confident of a diagnosis at the definite level even though the subject appears to have met the criteria. The designation of "clinical" or "possible" is most frequently used when there is insufficiently detailed information to meet the specified criteria and yet nevertheless the description of the episode(s) of illness appears "clinically" to be highly likely to have met those criteria.

The assignment of the conditions in Table 2–1 therefore, reflects one group's integration of the evidence from the literature regarding

TABLE 2-1
RDC Diagnostic Hierarchies for Genetic Studies of Bipolar Disorder

Each RDC disorder is classified as affected (A), uncertain (U), or not affected (N) given a particular set of hierarchical rules. The rules use the RDC categories as well as the levels of certainty of diagnosis: definite, probable, and clinical.

I. Narrowest System

Affected. Lifetime occurrence of a manic syndrome at the probable or definite level. This includes probable or definite bipolar I disorder and unipolar manic disorder, as well as the bipolar and manic forms of schizoaffective disorder.

Uncertain. All other major affective or schizoaffective disorders, hypomanic disorder and cyclothymic disorder, recurrent and chronic minor depressive disorder, intermittent depressive disorder, labile personality disorder, acute and subacute schizophrenic disorder, and unspecified psychosis.

Not affected. Single-episode minor depressive disorder and all other non-affective mental disorders, (including "other psychiatric disorder"), as well as never mentally ill.

II. Narrow System

Affected. Same as affected under system I, plus probable or definite bipolar II disorder with major depression, recurrent unipolar schizoaffective disorder (depression only), and recurrent unipolar major depressive disorder.

Uncertain. All other affective or schizoaffective disorders, including single-episode unipolar schizoaffective or major depressive disorder, bipolar II disorder with minor depression, unipolar hypomanic disorder, cyclothymic disorder, recurrent and chronic minor depressive disorder, intermittent depressive disorder, labile personality disorder, acute and subacute schizophrenic disorder, and unspecified psychosis.

Not affected. Same as under system I.

III. Broad System

Affected. Same as affected under systems I and II plus disorders with a manic syndrome at the clinical level (clinical bipolar I and unipolar manic disorders as well as the bipolar and manic forms of schizoaffective disorder); clinical-level bipolar II disorder with major depression; clinical-level recurrent unipolar schizoaffective disorder and recurrent unipolar major depressive disorder.

Uncertain. All other affective or schizoaffective disorders including single-episode unipolar schizoaffective or major depressive disorder, recurrent and chronic Minor depressive disorder, Intermittent depressive disorder, labile personality disorder, acute and subacute schizophrenic disorder, and unspecified psychosis.

Not affected. Same as systems I and II.

IV. Broadest System

Affected. Same as affected under systems I, II, and III plus all other disorders with hypomania or major depressive syndromes at the clinical, probable, or definite level. This will include unipolar hypomanic disorder, cyclothymic disorder, bipolar II disorder with minor depressive disorder, single-episode unipolar major depressive disorder, and schizoaffective depressive disorder.

Uncertain. Recurrent or chronic minor depressive disorder, Intermittent depressive disorder, labile personality disorder as well as probable level for "near hypomanic" periods, acute and subacute schizophrenic disorder, and unspecified psychosis.

Not affected. Same as systems I, II, and II.

TABLE 2–2
The Rates of "Affected" Subjects by Four Diagnostic Hierarchies

Pedigree	(N)	Narrowest I	Narrow II	Broad III	Broadest IV
A	(52)	8%	19%	21%	29%
B	(44)	9	39	39	52
C	(71)	6	27	31	49
D	(42)	21	38	43	57

the best placement for various disorders thought to be in the spectrum with bipolar I disorder, as well as the degree of certainty expressed by the diagnosticians for individual subjects within the pedigree.

Table 2–2 indicates the effects on the rates of affected of the different systems based on the data from four of the pedigrees in our current study. The effects are not of equal magnitude across all four pedigrees. For example, in pedigree A, the rates of affected vary from 8% to 29% (a little over a threefold increase), while in pedigree C, the change from 6% to 49% is an eightfold increase. Table 2–2 also indicates the difficulties of limiting the analyses to those subjects classified as affected by the narrowest system (level I) only. Only one of these four pedigrees (D) would have been very informative with that restriction. Most investigators would use the narrow system (level II) for their analyses if there are few subjects who meet the criteria for level I in the pedigree.

AN ALTERNATIVE TO THE USUAL DIAGNOSTIC HIERARCHIES

Using the diagnostic hierarchies as noted in Table 2–1 allows the investigator to take into account the certainty with which the clinician makes a particular diagnosis. However, each subject is still characterized dichotomously as affected or unaffected in the analyses of the data.

It may also be possible to convert the phenotypic descriptions into quantitative measures that take into account the clinical features, course of illness and even biological measures in some instances. Such as recurrence, age at onset, and severity as reflected in number of symptoms may be used to assign a likelihood weight to each case (Rice et al., 1986, 1987) or other studies that support the use of specific features to help define the degree to which the subject has a disorder that is more likely to be related to the core condition under study.

SUGGESTED PROCEDURES FOR OBTAINING DIAGNOSTIC DATA

Investigators have found that it is best to use all available sources of information for the diagnostic evaluations of all members of the pedigree, whether or not they are available for direct interview. This will often include interviews of the subject and as many family informants as can be obtained, review of medical records, and (when possible) interviews or discussions with current and past therapists or other nonfamily informants. The interviews and the review of records are guided by the particular sets of inclusion and exclusion criteria being used (see discussion of selection of criteria). Every effort should be made to clarify diagnostic issues with each informant. Whenever possible, there should be an option to return to the subject or an informant to seek clarification. Of course, those who are collecting diagnostic data should be "blind" with regard to biological marker data or results of linkage analyses. If possible, there should also be blindness with regard to familial relationship and affected status of other family members. It is often impossible and impractical to keep the interviewers totally blind with regard to these family factors; however, they must be kept blind as to laboratory findings.

Need for Experienced Clinicians

Unfortunately, when done well, the process of collecting good diagnostic information for genetic linkage studies of mental disorder is quite expensive. There is no easy or cheap way to obtain the valid diagnostic data in the extended families that are needed for these studies. The investigator should use experienced clinicians as the interviewers, abstractors of clinical records, and "consensus" diagnosticians. The clinicians should be very familiar with the specific diagnostic criteria being employed, as well as their intent. They should have considerable clinical experience with patients with the spectrum conditions of interest, as well as with the core disorder. The investigator should determine that each of the involved clinicians is aware of the major differential issues and is judging the items of specific information and using the criteria in a reliable fashion. When possible, formal reliability studies should be conducted prior to the actual data collection. In any case, senior supervisory clinicians should review the data as they are completed and quickly raise differential diagnostic issues or seek clarification at a time when it is easy to recontact the subject or the informant.

Interview Guides

The direct interviews with the subjects themselves and with the family informants should be semistructured clinical interviews with focused coverage, suggested questions, specific items of information to be scored, and some reminders of the differential diagnostic issues to be addressed. A number of such procedures are now available (see below), depending on the sets of diagnostic criteria being used in a particular study. Regardless of the specific structured procedure used, the clinician should be free to follow up on seeming contradictions in the subject's reports, inconsistencies, and any clinical insights that occur during the process of the interview. Special care should be taken to ascertain that the intent of a particular item is indeed met before it is scored as positive.

The major potential disadvantages of the use of structured clinical interviews include the pseudoendorsement of the items, lack of coverage of some clinical concepts, and dulled attention on the part of the interviewer to important differential diagnostic issues. To avoid the pseudoendorsement of items, the interviewer should always obtain and record examples of the behavior or symptoms in question before scoring the item present. If the clinician conducting the interview knows the intent of the items, the likelihood is much lower that they will be falsely endorsed. If the structured interview guide selected for use in the study does not cover some of the clinical concepts considered to be of importance by the investigator, it should be supplemented with additional suggested questions and items. Some investigators hope the clinicians will attend to the extra coverage and will address the issues in their narratives. Unfortunately, in the absence of reminders in the form of questions and items, many of the them will fail to do so. Interviewers who are not called upon to make their own summary diagnostic judgments after the evaluation is completed are much more likely to use the guide in a routine fashion and to pay less attention to the differential diagnostic issues that arise with a particular subject. Some investigators are reluctant to request the interviewers to make diagnostic judgments for fear that it will somehow prejudice the evaluation. Given that it is unlikely that a clinician will conduct an evaluation without gaining some diagnostic impression, it is far better that the recording of that impression be done in a systematic fashion and that there be an awareness of the need for such judgments at the end of the evaluation. Such attention will also help focus the interview and the follow-up questions.

SUGGESTED GUIDELINES FOR OBTAINING SUMMARY OR CONSENSUS DIAGNOSTIC EVALUATIONS

Eventually an investigator will have obtained varying amounts of diagnostic data for each of the subjects in the pedigree—but unfortunately, there is no simple way to combine the data into the most correct diagnosis. Usually one or more senior clinicians are used as "best estimate" diagnosticians. Obviously, these consensus or "best-estimate consensus" diagnosticians should be blind to family relationships and to any laboratory or biological markers that have been identified. Ideally, at least two independent diagnosticians would review the materials for each subject and make independent best-estimate diagnoses. Any disagreements that are not readily settled between the two independent diagnosticians should be resolved after a third senior diagnostician completes another independent review of the same materials. At times, the agreement will be that no agreement can be reached regarding a particular diagnosis, age at onset, and so on. All subjects about whom there has been diagnostic disagreement, and further discussion or the use of an additional rater, should be "tagged" because this is an indication that there was something about the subject or the available data that raised diagnostic questions. At times, it may be possible to recontact the subject or an informant to clarify some issues, but often this cannot be done.

The consensus diagnosticians should be provided with specific items of information on the phenomenology of all episodes of the illness, course of the illness, degree of impairment and residual symptoms between episodes, and any specific problems that might be related to differential diagnostic issues. They should obtain narrative descriptions from the various clinical interviews with a focus on the syndromal nature of all detected conditions, the timing of their onsets and offsets (particularly relative to each other), and their longitudinal course. Any conditions or situational variables that may have compromised the validity of the data available (e.g., denial, presence of a child or spouse in the room) or any complicated clinical features (e.g., possible head injury or organic brain syndrome) should be noted in the materials given to the consensus diagnosticians.

The consensus diagnosticians should have some agreed-upon rules for combining information from different sources and rules for indicating the level of clinical certainty with which they make their diagnostic judgments. Subjects should be tagged for atypical clinical features. All of the diagnostic judgments and tagging of subjects should be done before any linkage analyses are run. Such tagging not only should include unusual clinical features and diagnostic difficulties, but also deviations from the classical clinical features.

SELECTION OF CRITERIA AND EVALUATION PROCEDURES

Given our current state of knowledge, or lack thereof, about the best critera sets for the diagnosis of specific mental disorders, it behooves the investigator who is conducting a study of the genetics of mental disorders to collect the data needed for the application of more than one diagnostic "system." Furthermore, the investigator should make sure to collect sufficient details in the symptom descriptions to be able to apply new sets of criteria as they are developed or proposed. In addition, if certain clinical features are thought to be important, they should be collected even if they are not part of any of the critera sets generally applied. If the investigator has some evidence that particular clinical features frequently appear to be associated with the disorder of interest in some families, it is important to try to collect similar data for all families. Such clinical features may later be of value in describing linked and unlinked families for a particular type of genetic linkage. Anger dyscontrol is an example of such clinical features and artistic creativity is another.

The two sets of diagnostic criteria most commonly used in the United States for the study of major affective disorders are the Research Diagnostic Criteria (RDC) (Spitzer, Endicott, & Robins, 1978) and the various editions of the *Diagnostic and Statistical Manual Mental Disorders* (DSM-III, DSM-III-Revised) of the American Psychiatric Association. Fortunately, there is fairly good agreement between these two systems, although there are some differences that can have major implications regarding the placement of a disorder within a particular hierarchical system for classifying affected, uncertain, and unaffected subjects. For example, there are differences with regard to the differential diagnosis of schizoaffective disorder from manic and major depressive disorders that can have effects even at the narrow (level II) classification mentioned previously.

The procedure most commonly used to collect the information needed for the RDC is the lifetime version of the Schedule for Affective Disorders and Schizophrenia (Endicott & Spitzer, 1978) modified for bipolar disorders (SADS-LB). The Family History–Research Diagnostic Criteria (FH-RDC) are designed for use in interviewing family informants or others who know the subject well (Andreasen, Endicott, Spitzer, & Winokur, 1977). Both of these procedures focus on episodes of syndromal disorder that are then further subtyped for current disorders and past disorders. Ages at onset and number of recurrences are also noted, as are the specific symptoms manifested. The procedure most commonly used for DSM-III diagnoses is the Structured Clinical Interview for Diagnosis (SCID) (Spitzer, Williams, Gibbon, & First, 1990). More recently, the National Institute of Mental Health (NIMH) developed new procedures referred to as the Diagnostic Interview for Genetic Studies (DIGS) and the Family Interview for Genetic Studies (FIGS). These two procedures will be used in the NIMH Diagnostic Centers for Psychiatric Linkage Studies that are focused on schizophrenia and bipolar spectrum disorders.

As more is learned about bipolar disorders and other affective disorders, the procedures to collect data and the criteria themselves will undoubtedly change. Investigators who are currently involved in or are planning such studies should familiarize themselves with the procedures currently in use and those being developed, and make informed decisions regarding the criteria to be used and the data to be recorded.

REFERENCES

Andreasen, N. C., Endicott, J., Spitzer, R. L., & Winokur, G. (1977). The family history method using diagnostic criteria. *Archives of General Psychiatry, 34,* 1229–1235.

Baron, M., & Endicott, J. (1990). Genetic linkage in mental illness: Limitations and prospects. *British Journal Psychiatry, 157,* 645–655.

Baron, M., Hamburger, R., Sanduyl, L. A., Risch, N., Mandel, B., Endicott, J., Belmaker, R. H., & Ott, J. (1990). The impact of phenotypic variation on genetic analysis: Application to x-linkage in manic-depressive illness. *Acta Psychiatrica Scandinavica, 82,* 196–203.

Coryell, W., Endicott, J., Andreasen, N. C., & Keller M. (1985). Bipolar I, bipolar II, and nonbipolar major depression among the relatives of affectively ill probands. *American Journal of Psychiatry, 142* (7), 817–821.

Coryell, W., Endicott, J., Reich, T., Andreasen, N., & Keller, M. B. (1984). A family study of bipolar II disorder. *British Journal of Psychiatry, 145,* 49–54.

Coryell, W., Keller, M., Endicott, J., & Andreasen, N. (1989). Bipolar II illness: Course and outcome over a 5-year period. *Psychological Medicine 19,* 129–141.

Detre, T., Himmelhoch, J., Schwartzburg, M., Anderson, C. M., Byck, R., & Kupfer, D. J. (1972). Hypersomnia and manic-depressive disease. *American Journal of Psychiatry, 128,* 1303–1305.

Egeland, J. A., Sussex, J. N., Endicott, J., Hostetter, A. M., Offord, R. D., Schwab, J. J., Allen, C. R., & Pauls, D. L. (1991). Impact of diagnoses on genetic linkage study for bipolar affective disorders among the Amish. *Journal of Psychiatric Genetics, 1,* 5–18.

Endicott, J., Nee, J., Andreasen, N., Clayton, P., Keller, M., & Coryell, W. (1985). Bipolar II: Combine or keep separate? *J Aff. Dis., 8,* 17–28.

Endicott, J., Nee, J., Coryell, W., Andreasen, N., & Croughan, J. (1986). Schizoaffective, psychotic, and nonpsychotic depression: Differential familial association. *Comprehensive Psychiatry 27,* 1–13.

Endicott, J., & Spitzer, R. L. (1978). A diagnostic interview: The Schedule for Affective Disorders and Schizophrenia. *Archives of General Psychiatry, 35,* 837–844.

Gershon, E. S., Hamovit, S., Guroff, J. J., Dibble, E., Leckman, J. F., Sceery, W., Targun, S. D., Nurnberger, J. F., Goldin, L. R., & Bunney, W. E. (1982). A family study of schizoaffective, bipolar I, bipolar II, unipolar, and normal control probands. *Archives of General Psychiatry, 39,* 1157–1167.

Merikangas, K. R., Spenec, A., & Kupfer, D. J. (1989). Linkage studies of bipolar disorder: Methodologic and analytic issues. *Archives of General Psychiatry, 46,* 1137–1141.

Rice, J., Endicott, J., Knesevich, M. A., & Rochberg, N. J. (1987). The estimation of diagnostic sensitivity using stability data: An application to major depressive disorder. *Journal of Psychiatry Research, 21,* 337–346.

Rice, J. P., McDonald-Scott, P., Endicott, J., Coryell, W., Grove, W. M., Keller, M. B., & Altis, D. (1986). The stability of diagnosis with an application to bipolar II disorder. *Journal of Psychiatry Research, 19,* 285–296.

Rice, J. P., Reich, T., Andreasen, N., Coryell, W., & Endicott, J. (1984). Validity of the bipolar/unipolar dichotomy. *CI Neuropharmacol, 7* (Suppl 1), 716–717.

Rice, J., Reich, T., Andreasen, N. C., Endicott, J., Van Eerdewegh, M., Fishman, R., Hirschfeld, R. M. A., & Klerman, G. L. (1987). The familial transmission of bipolar illness. *Archives of General Psychiatry, 44,* 441–447.

Spitzer, R. L., Endicott, J., & Robins, E. (1978). Research Diagnostic Criteria: Rationale and reliability. *Archives of General Psychiatry, 35,* 773–782.

Spitzer, R. L., Williams, J. B. W., Gibbon, M., & First, M. B. (1990). *SCID user's guide for the structured clinical interview for DSM-III-R.* Washington, DC: *American Psychiatric Press.*

3

Basic Principles in Linkage Analysis

HERBERT M. LACHMAN

Since the beginning of the recombinant DNA era in the mid-1970s, thousands of genes have been isolated and their DNA sequences determined. This has resulted in an unprecedented information explosion that has revolutionized our understanding of basic biological processes. Abnormalities in the genes involved in the development of cancer have been identified (Bishop, 1991), and the genes responsible for Duchenne's muscular dystrophy and cystic fibrosis have been cloned (Rommens et al., 1989; Kerem et al., 1989; Monaro et al., 1986). Furthermore, studies at the molecular genetic level have resulted in the discovery of an unprecedented number of novel neurotransmitter receptors. At the time of this writing, the first "gene therapy" is underway for a rare inherited immune abnormality, adenosine deaminase (ADA) deficiency. It can be argued that the recombinant DNA era will be viewed as spawning one of the most important scientific advances in human history. But despite these extraordinary successes, little progress has been made in understanding the fundamental molecular and genetic bases of inherited psychiatric disorders.

Why has understanding the biology of mental illness lagged behind other medical and scientific arenas? Perhaps the foremost reason is the complexity of the human brain, which is the most intricate biological structure in nature. Another obvious problem is the inaccessibility of

---

The Program in Behavioral Genetics is supported by the Ruane Family Fund and the G. Harold and Leila Y. Mathers charitable foundation. The author is a fellow of the Irma T. Hirschl and Monique Weill-Caulier Charitable Trust. He would also like to acknowledge Dr. Herman van Praag for his encouragement and support in establishing the Program of Behavioral Genetics.

the brain to experimental manipulation. As a result, most studies of psychiatric disorders are descriptive and phenomenological. While these can be very interesting, many of the observed changes appear to be state dependent and, therefore may not address underlying pathophysiology at the level of the central nervous system (CNS). This is particularly the case in studies of depressed patients that examine neurotransmitter receptors expressed in peripheral tissue, such as lymphocytes and platelets (Berrettini, Cappellari, & Gershon, 1987). Third, there are no reliable biological markers of depression or mania that would serve to differentiate between the asymptomatic carriers of an abnormal gene and normal individuals who are not carriers, a critical consideration for genetic analysis. Finally, the genetic tools available for the isolation of the genes that are responsible for inherited conditions rely heavily on the presence of a single dominant genetic locus as well as on unequivocal diagnostic criteria. (These issues are addressed in Chapters 2 and 5.) For those interested in exploring the underlying molecular and genetic basis of inherited psychiatric conditions, nature has not been a willing collaborator.

This chapter reviews the methods used by investigators to identify genes involved in inherited conditions. In particular, it focuses on linkage analysis, a method of gene mapping that is being applied to determine the location of the chromosomal region that may contain genes that predispose an individual to manic-depressive disorder. The aim is to provide the reader with a scientific and historical framework to help understand the unique complexities involved in the study of inherited psychiatric conditions.

STRUCTURE OF DNA

The structure of DNA is a model of elegant simplicity. Its fundamental subunit is the nucleotide base, which consists of a simple nitrogen-containing ring structure attached to a 5-carbon sugar group called deoxyribose and a phosphate group. DNA is made up of long chains of these nucleotide bases attached by a phosphodiester linkage formed between the phosphate group of one nucleotide and the deoxyribose of the adjacent nucleotide. Essentially, only four principal nucleotide bases (or slight modifications thereof) constitute the genomes of every living entity on the planet: guanine (G), adenine (A), thymine (T), and cytosine (C). Most DNA molecules, with the exception of certain viruses, are double stranded, with the sequences of one strand bound to the second by hydrogen bonds formed between the nucleotide bases. The DNA sequence of the second strand is uniquely determined by the sequences of the first strand. Within the sterical restriction of the double-stranded DNA molecule, hydrogen bonds can only be formed between specific complementary nucleotide bases: C binds to G on the opposite strands and A binds to T, a process called base pairing. Consequently, the nucleotide sequence CTGTTCGAAGT on one strand requires that the complementary strand have the corresponding sequence GACAAGCTTCA to form the double-stranded structure:

CTGTTCGAAGT
GACAAGCTTCA

When DNA replicates during cell division, the strands separate and nucleotides are added to the single-stranded DNA molecules. It is not difficult to visualize that this process will lead to the formation of two exact replicas of the original double-stranded DNA molecule.

Double-stranded DNA is folded in a spiral array that is referred to as the "double helix." The discovery of base pairing and the double helical structure of native DNA by Watson and Crick in 1953, based on the x-ray crystallographs prepared by Franklin and Wilkins, solved the greatest mystery in biology. This knowledge launched a series of discoveries that led to the elucidation of the fundamental processes of life—the mechanism of cell division and the remarkable process that decodes DNA into RNA and protein. In the current era of multiauthor, multi-institution publications and the emergence of hundreds of new journals to handle the biological information explosion, it is noteworthy that the landmark paper reporting the double helical structure of DNA, which inaugurated the modern biological era, appeared as a single page in a 1953 issue of the journal *Nature* (Watson & Crick, 1953).

The entire human genome consists of approximately three billion nucleotide base pairs, which are found in every nucleated somatic cell. This number is about 1,000-fold greater than the amount of DNA found in a bacterium, but only half as much as that found in *Rana pipiens,* a frog. The order of the nucleotide bases determines the structure of specific genes. Nucleotides, therefore, are analogous to the letters of a word with each gene containing hundreds and thousands of "letters." Genes are decoded (transcribed) into a single-stranded RNA precurser that is an exact replica of one of the DNA strands, except that the sugar moiety consists of ribose instead of deoxyribose. In addition, RNA and DNA differ in that a nucleotide equivalent called uracil substitutes for thymine in RNA. The precursor RNA is converted into a messenger RNA (mRNA) molecule by a series of processing reactions. It is not within the scope of this review to discuss these molecular events. The interested reader is referred to the text *Molecular Cell Biology* (Darnell, Lodish, & Baltimore, 1990).

Messenger RNA is transported to ribosomes, the protein-synthesizing factories of the cell located in the cytosol, where it is "translated" into a protein. Every three continuous nucleotide bases represented on the DNA and mRNA, called a codon, encode for a specific amino-acid residue. Starting at a specific "start" signal, the mRNA is translated into a protein, the amino-acid sequence of which is predetermined by the order of codons that is found on the gene. Translation continues through the mRNA until a "stop" signal is reached. Mutations in the DNA sequence of a gene could result in a change in the amino-acid sequence of its encoded protein. A single mutation in a gene could have profound consequences for an individual. For example, a change in the sixth codon of the a-globin gene resulting in the substitution of a leucine amino-acid residue for glutamic acid leads to sickle cell anemia. This disease results in severe anemia and causes painful ischemic events in the bones, debilitation, and early death. The power of such a single "point mutation" occurring in a genome that contains three billion nucleotides is analogous to a typographical error's completely altering the meaning of an encyclopedia.

DNA is tightly consolidated in the nucleus by various proteins, such as histones. Packaged protein-bound DNA is referred to as chromatin. If one were to remove the chromatin proteins and unwind the DNA from a single human cell, it would stretch approximately 3 feet. During cell division, DNA is duplicated and partitioned into chromosomes. Each somatic cell in humans contains 22 pairs of chromosomes and two sex chromosomes, 46 altogether, which include the 100,000 genes that are thought to constitute the human genome.

BASIC RECOMBINANT DNA

Although the techniques used to identify novel genes may take several years to master, the entire recombinant DNA process can be simplified into three fundamental steps. First, DNA can be cut across the double-stranded structure using a series of enzymes called restriction endonucleases (Meselson & Yuan, 1968; Smith, 1979). These enzymes are derived from microorganisms, and so far, hundreds have been purified and are commercially available. Each restriction enzyme recognizes unique short sequences of double-stranded DNA, so that DNA will be cleaved across the double helix wherever the recognition sequences appear (Figure 3–1). The size of the DNA fragments generated by restriction endonuclease digestion depends on the distance between successive recognition sites. For simple DNA molecules, such as the DNA that constitutes the genome of bacterial plasmids, restriction digestion results in a small number of different DNA fragments. However, human DNA is much more complex. Restriction endonuclease digestion may cleave human DNA into tens of thousands of pieces. Since the distance between successive restriction endonuclease recognition sites is not fixed, the sizes of the multitude of DNA fragments generated by restriction endonuclease digestion will be randomly distributed.

The second fundamental principle is that the individual strands that constitute DNA can be separated (denatured or melted) upon heating it at 95°, and the complementary strands can be reannealed upon cooling, thereby restoring the original double-stranded configuration. An important variation of this process occurs when two sources of DNA are melted and reannealed together. If the DNA from source A has sufficient sequence similarity to that from source B, then unique, reannealed double-stranded DNA sequences can be formed. If one source of DNA is denatured and fixed to a DNA binding filter and another is radiolabeled by one of several simple labeling strategies and denatured, unique reannealed DNA sequences can be formed by mixing the probe with the filters and visualized by exposing the filter to sensitive x-ray film. The process of annealing DNA from two different sources is referred to as hybridization and forms the primary basis for gene identification.

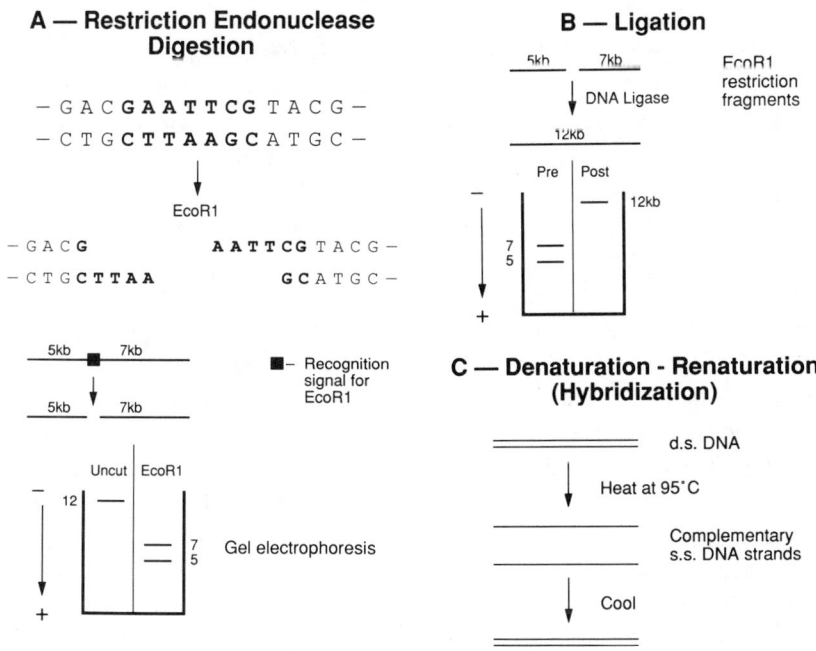

Figure 3–1(A). Restriction endonuclease digestion. The double-stranded recognition signal for the enzyme *EcoR1* is shown in boldface. Cleavage will generate two double-stranded molecules that contain single-stranded termini. Note that these termini are complementary to each other. A linear piece of DNA that is 12 kb in length will be cleaved into two smaller fragments according to the position of the *EcoR1* recognition signal (not drawn to scale). The different DNA fragments obtained before and after digestion can be resolved by gel electrophoresis, a technique that separates DNA fragments in an electric field according to size.

(B). Ligation. Two DNA fragments with compatible complementary ends, such as the *EcoR1* digested DNA fragments shown in Figure 3–1(A), can be reattached using the enzyme DNA ligase. The electrophoresis pattern shows the different fragments pre- and post-ligation.

(C). Hybridization. Double-stranded (d.s.) DNA can be separated into single-stranded (s.s.) strands by heat. The strands can be reannealed to the original ds structure upon cooling.

The third principle is that restriction-digested DNA, or other appropriately generated DNA fragments, can be reattached using enzymes called "ligases." These enzymes attach double-stranded DNA molecules by catalyzing the phosphodiester linkage that forms the DNA backbone. There is no species specificity to ligation reactions. Consequently, a piece of restriction-digested human DNA can be ligated to a similarly cut DNA fragment derived from any other source, such as bacterial plasmids or viruses. Plasmids are autonomously replicating DNA elements that "infect" certain strains of bacteria and are responsible for conferring bacterial antibiotic resistance. One can grow reiterated copies of any fragment of DNA by ligating it into a plasmid and isolating clones of antibiotic-resistant bacteria infected with the plasmid. Novel DNA fragments generated in this way are called recombinants. One can also generate recombinants using bacteriophage, a family of viruses that infect bacteria. The growth of recombinant plasmids or bacteriophage-containing ligated genes of interest is referred to as cloning. This strategy essentially allows an investigator to isolate very large quantities of a particular gene or DNA segment.

CREATING A DNA LIBRARY

The basic strategy for cloning new genes utilizes all of these fundamental concepts. Suppose that a gene that encodes a particular neurotransmitter receptor gene derived from rodent DNA has been identified and an investigator is interested in cloning the homolog of that gene in human DNA. The first step is to create a "library" of human DNA. There are two types of libraries—"genomic," which is derived from the DNA extracted from any source of nucleated cells, and "cDNA," which is derived from RNA using tissue in which the gene of interest is likely to be expressed. For example, if one is interested in cloning a neurotransmitter receptor gene, brain RNA or RNA derived from a neuronal cell line would be an appropriate source of tissue. Purified mRNA is converted into DNA (complementary or cDNA) using the enzymes reverse transcriptase and DNA polymerase. Complementary DNA is then ligated into bacteriophage DNA.

In the generation of genomic libraries, cellular DNA is first digested with an appropriate restriction enzyme and then ligated into the DNA of a similarly digested plasmid or bacteriophage (Sambrook, Fritsch, & Maniatis, 1989). For a variety of reasons, cDNA libraries have a number of advantages, although genomic libraries have uses that cannot be ascribed to cDNA, such as cloning regions near a gene that are involved in regulating its expression, but do not appear in the mRNA. The plasmid or bacteriophage library is used to infect appropriate strains of bacteria, which are then grown on agar plates. After 8–12 hours in an incubator, individual colonies representing the growth from a single infected bacterium containing a unique DNA fragment from the library appear on the plate (Figure 3–2). In a typical experiment, 10 to 20 plates of bacteria, each containing 10,000–50,000 colonies, are grown, ensuring that most of the genome is analyzed. After incubation, the colonies are transferred to a piece of DNA binding filter paper by placing the filter over the bacterial plate. After a few minutes of contact, a fraction of the bacteria from each individual colony adheres to the filter paper and another fraction remains on the plate. The filter and plate are oriented with respect to each other by marking both at the same positions with indelible ink. The DNA from the filter-bound bacterial colonies is exposed and denatured by treating the filters with detergent and strong alkali respectively.

In order to identify the recombinant plasmid or bacteriophage of interest in a background of up to one to two million negative recombinants, a sensitive hybridization analysis is performed in which the filters are treated with radiolabeled copies of specific and selective single-stranded DNA or RNA probes that have sequence similarity to the gene of interest, in this example, the neurotransmitter receptor gene derived from rats. Since the DNA sequence of individual genes is well conserved between species, some of the radiolabeled probe will anneal to homologous sequences in the human recombinant library. Following a period of 8–12 hours, the filters are washed and dried to remove nonspecifically bound probe, and are then exposed to x-ray film for approximately 24 hours. Positive signals will be observed on developed films corresponding to the recombinant plasmids or bacteriophages that specifically bind to the probe by virtue of their partial homology to each other. By orienting the film, filter, and bacterial plate, the original bacterial colony containing the specific recombinant plasmid or bacteriophage can be isolated, placed in a growth

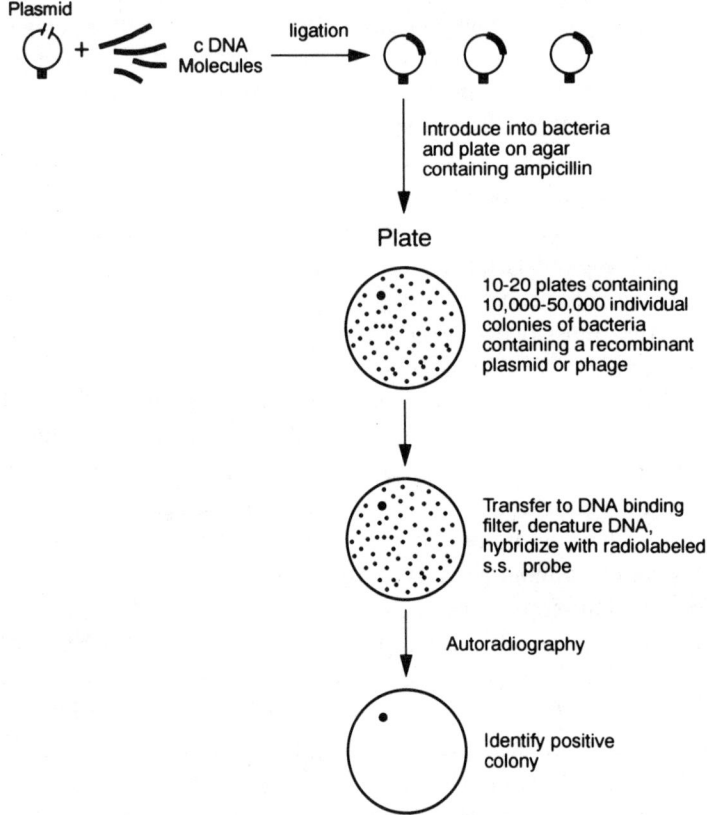

Figure 3–2. Cloning. Total cellular RNA is extracted from cells and is converted into complementary DNA (cDNA) using the enzyme reverse transcriptase (not shown). Complementary DNA is ligated into a bacteriophage or plasmid that has been opened with an appropriate restriction enzyme (for simplicity only, the plasmid example is shown). This generates a library of different recombinant plasmids, with each plasmid carrying a unique cDNA insert. The plasmid also contains a gene for antibiotic resistance—in this example, ampicillin (solid box on plasmid)—such that bacteria infected with the plasmid will grow on ampicillin-containing agar plates. Colonies of ampicillin-resistant bacteria infected with recombinant plasmids are grown. The colonies are partially transferred to DNA binding filters and the DNA within the bacteria is released and denatured into single strands. The gene of interest is identified by hybridizing the filters with radiolabeled complementary single-stranded DNA or RNA probes. Autoradiography identifies the small number of recombinant plasmids that actually contain the gene of interest. The bacteria containing this plasmid can be recovered from the original plate and grown in large quantities.

medium, and expanded. Subsequently, large quantities of the gene of interest can be isolated from the bacteria and then characterized by DNA sequence analysis and tissue expression. In addition to obtaining DNA, functional protein, encoded by a full-length gene insert, can also be obtained by using certain plasmid or bacteriophage vectors that support eukaryotic gene expression. This very abridged version of a cloning experiment corresponds to the work of one postdoctoral fellow or graduate student working full time for approximately a year.

Another cloning strategy involves the same basic technique, except that, instead of screening with labeled DNA or RNA probes, immunological methods are employed. Libraries that express eukaryotic proteins derived from gene inserts can be probed with specific antibodies directed against the protein encoded by the gene of interest. This technique is used if one has successfully generated an antibody to the purified protein.

Unfortunately, these strategies cannot be used as a first step to identify potential target genes that predispose to manic-depressive disorder because there are, as yet, no reliable biological markers for the illness. In heritable conditions in which a direct cloning of the gene of interest is not possible, an important method of investigation involves identifying the chromosomal location of the unknown gene by a technique referred to as linkage analysis.

LINKAGE ANALYSIS

As a first step in cloning unknown genes, it is critical to identify the chromosomal fragment that contains the gene of interest using a technique called linkage analysis. The fundamental concept of linkage is that if two traits are inherited together but are encoded by different genes, the genes will be found in the same chromosomal region. In other words, if trait A is known to be caused by a gene on chromosome 9, and trait B is associated with a clinically recognized syndrome but neither the gene nor its chromosomal position is known, coinheritance of traits A and B would suggest that the gene causing trait B is also on chromosome 9. If traits A and B separate (segregate) in a pedigree such that many individuals have either trait A or trait B, the genes cannot be physically linked to the same chromosomal region.

In order to illustrate how linkage analysis is accomplished, the terms "homologous chromosome" and "allele" must be explained. With the exception of the sex chromosomes, every somatic cell contains two copies of every chromosome, referred to as homologous chromosomes, one inherited from the mother and the other from the father. Each homologous chromosome pair has precisely the same gene order. Thus there are two copies of every gene on all somatic cells.

The copies of similar genes found on homologous chromosomes are referred to as alleles. The allelic copies of genes often have precisely the same DNA sequence. This is especially true for genes that encode proteins with very specialized, invariant functions, such as those that encode the protein portion of hemoglobin. However, in traits associated with variability in the population that are not associated with strong evolutionary selective advantage, such as eye and hair color, alleles may differ slightly in their DNA sequence.

A variation in the DNA sequence between individuals is referred to as a polymorphism. Allelic differences can result in inherited disorders if the change in the encoded protein is deleterious. Polymorphisms are very useful for linkage analysis if present in a fairly substantial portion of the population (5–10%). For example, red–green color blindness is a polymorphic trait located on the long arm of the X chromosome that is present in almost 10% of the male population. Consequently, in a family carrying a particular genetic defect as well as color blindness, one could assign the defect to a gene on the X chromosome, if co-segregation with color blindness is found in a statistically significant number of male individuals in the family (for X-linked recessive conditions, only males are affected). Similarly, one can assign linkage to a particular chromosome using polymorphic traits associated with biochemical changes that can be easily assayed. For example, the gene encoding the enzyme glucose 6-phosphate dehydrogenase (G6PD) is known to be located on the X chromosome. G6PD is polymorphic in the population, resulting in the capacity of certain individuals to express two different isozymes that can be identified in the laboratory. In a family that transmits alleles for two different G6PD isozymes, one can assign an inherited condition to a gene on the X chromosome, if a number of individuals coinherit one particular G6PD isozyme, as well as the heritable illness.

Another example of a polymorphic locus that has been used in linkage analysis is the histocompatability human leukocyte antigen (HLA) region on chromosome 6, which is involved in T-lymphocyte–mediated immunity. The HLA locus is made up of dozens of genes that are highly polymorphic in the population. Linkage to chromosome 6 could be established if a genetic abnormality were found to be associated with specific HLA polymorphisms (haplotypes). Linkage to the HLA locus illustrates an important concept in linkage analysis: is the marker exclusively linked to a gene causing an inherited illness, or does it directly influence or cause the illness? For most markers, linkage is entirely circumstantial. However, a number of conditions linked to the HLA locus are autoimmune, such as ankylosing spondylitis, which is associated with the HLA-B27 haplotype. In these conditions, the HLA polymorphism is causally associated with pathogenesis.

One problem associated with all forms of linkage analysis is genetic recombination. During meiosis, the process that results in the formation of germ cells (ova and sperm), the 23 pairs of homologous chromosomes randomly segregate in such a way that each daughter cell contains single copies of the 23 chromosomes. The full chromosomal complement is restored at fertilization. During meiosis, a free exchange of genetic material occurs, in an equal and reciprocal fashion, between homologous chromosomes. This process is referred to as recombination. As a result of recombination, the chromosomes that segregate during meiosis are actually chimeras of maternal and paternal genetic material. The recombination frequency is proportional to the genetic distance between two genes and is approximately 1% for every one million nucleotides. Recombination that occurs between a marker and a linked allele will result in the loss of linkage. Consequently, in a larger pedigree found to have a chromosome specific marker linked to a particular genetic illness located five million nucleotides away, approximately 5% of affected individuals will not have the "correct" linkage pattern (Figure 3–3). Furthermore, in a chromosome containing 100 million nucleotides, two genes located on opposite ends would essentially segregate as if they were on different chromosomes. Therefore, in order to establish linkage, the marker polymorphic trait and the allele causing a genetic illness must be in relatively close proximity on a particular chromosomal segment, usually within 10 million

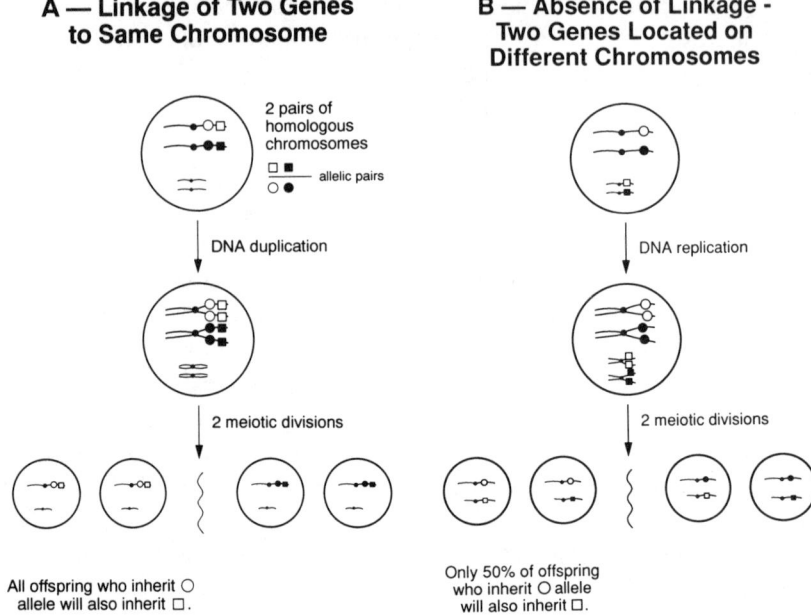

Figure 3–3(A). Linkage of two genes to same chromosome. Two sets of homologous chromosomes are shown with two allelic gene pairs. The open and solid circles constitute one gene pair and the open and solid squares the other (the central small solid circle is the centromere of the chromosome). The alleles differ in their DNA sequence such that each gene encodes a different recognizable phenotype (closed versus open configuration). Assume that the open circle encodes a mutant allele that results in an inherited illness and the open square enocodes a marker phenotype, such as brown eyes (the solid circle therefore would represent the normal allele and the open circle a different eye color). In this example, a parent is heterozygous for both genes (contains one copy of each allele). During meiosis, which generates germ cells, the different homologous chromosomes segregate. Since the mutant allele is on the same homologous chromosome as the marker allele, the germ cells generated during meiosis will retain the linkage. Consequently, all of the offspring who inherit the marker open square allele also inherit the open circle mutant allele.

(B). Absence of linkage. If the marker and mutant alleles are located on separate chromosomes, they will randomly segregate during meiosis. In this example, there is only a 50% probability that offspring who inherit the marker open square will also inherit the mutant allele.

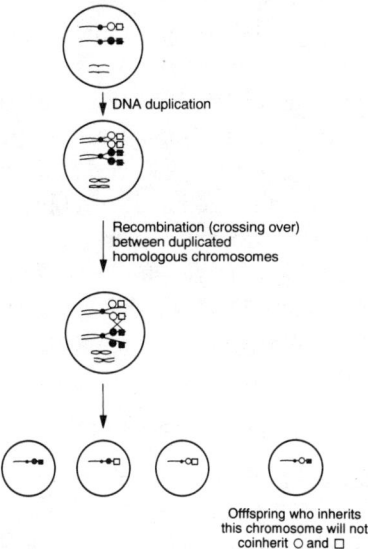

Figure 3-3. *(Continued)*
(C). Recombination. Even though two genes are on same chromosome, their linkage may be lost through recombination. During meiosis, an equal exchange of material takes place between homologous chromosomes. If this occurs between the marker and mutant allele, the linkage between the two will be lost. Therefore, an individual who inherits a recombinant chromosome will inherit the mutant open circle along with a solid square, which does not encode the marker phenotype. The recombination frequency is proportional to genetic distance. If the marker allele and mutant allele are one million bases apart, then one would expect that approximately 1/100 meiotic episodes would result in a germ cell that does show linkage (for simplicity, only one meiosis is shown).

nucleotides of each other. Moreover, large pedigrees are often required to establish linkage, particularly for markers that are relatively far from the gene of interest.

The concepts of linkage and chromosomal recombination are shown in Figures 3–3(A–C).

Relying on polymorphic differences that are based on either a biochemical assay or a specific physical trait is a limitation since the probability of finding such a marker linked to a gene of interest is relatively low. However, the probability of establishing linkage dramatically increases by using polymorphic markers that are easily detected and randomly distributed in large numbers. These criteria are precisely what the recombinant DNA era has provided in the form of restriction fragment length polymorphisms (RFLPs).

RFLP ANALYSIS

Of the estimated three billion nucleotide base pairs found in the genome, approximately 5% encode specific genes. The remaining 95%, which constitute the intergenic regions, are euphemistically referred to as "junk DNA," and have no well-established function. Since intergenic DNA does not encode any specific gene product, there is less evolutionary pressure to conserve specific DNA sequences in these regions among individuals. Consequently, the sequence of a random piece of intergenic DNA will differ slightly among individuals in the population, perhaps of the order of 1%. Since recognition sites for the hundreds of known restriction endonuclease enzymes are randomly distributed across the genome and occur on the average of once every few hundred nucleotide base pairs, it is not uncommon that a polymorphism will be found at a restriction endonuclease recognition site. Since the affinity of a restriction enzyme for its DNA recognition site is relatively strong, a single base difference will usually prevent endonuclease binding, thereby precluding DNA digestion at that site. In addition, it is also possible that a random mutation will create a new recognition site for a particular restriction endonuclease that did not previously exist.

When human DNA is digested with restriction endonucleases, thousands of individual pieces are generated. However, if there are polymorphic sites that create new restriction recognition signals or obliterate preexisting ones, the DNA fragments that are generated by a specific restriction endonuclease digestion will contain several distinctively sized fragments in certain individuals. These differences are detectable by a DNA analysis called Southern blotting. In this technique, restriction digested DNA is separated according to size by gel electrophoresis, denatured in alkali, and transferred to DNA binding filters. Following hybridization with radiolabeled single-stranded DNA or RNA probes, signals are generated on x-ray film corresponding to the binding of the probe to similar sequences in the genome. The size of the DNA fragments detected depends on the restriction enzyme used, as well as on the type of probe used. DNA probes derived from various chromosomes can be used to detect region-specific restriction fragments. Differences in the size of the DNA bands due to restriction polymorphisms are referred to as restriction fragment length polymorphisms, or RFLPs.

Another polymorphism identified by recombinant DNA techniques relies on the variability in the length of tandem repetitive DNA elements (VNTR). Repetitive DNA is an expanse of sequences that are reiterated a number of times throughout the genome. It may be randomly positioned on different chromosomes or arranged sequentially in a tandem array. Tandem repetitive elements are highly polymorphic with respect to the number of times the basic unit repeats itself in a particular chromosomal region. For example, one individual may have a repetitive element reiterated 10 times, whereas another may have 15 elements. Digestion of DNA with a restriction endonuclease that flanks the tandem repetitive site will result in restriction fragments that vary in size according to the number of repetitive units contained within the fragment.

In 1980, it was suggested that DNA polymorphisms causing RFLPs could be exploited for mapping genes to specific chromosomal regions (Botstein, White, Skolnick, & Davis, 1980). The idea was that a map could be generated by localizing numerous RFLPs to specific chromosomal regions. Then linkage of unknown genes could be established by a statistically significant association occurring between a mutant allele causing a particular inherited illness and a chromosome-specific RFLP. To illustrate, suppose that the location of an unknown gene is suspected to be located on a particular chromosome and a particular probe detects a 5-(kilobase, 1000 nucleotides) fragment in the region of interest following digestion with the restriction enzyme *EcoR1* (Figure 3–4). A polyphorism is found in a number of individuals that results in the loss of recognition for *EcoR1* at that particular site. In these individuals, the probe will detect a 12-kb fragment (note that the probe and detected fragments do not have to overlap over the entire distance of the DNA band in order to be detected). Since the RFLP is relatively rare, most individuals will be heterozygous; that is, one chromosome will contain the 5-kb band and its homologous partner the 12-kb band.

Say that an investigator finds that every member of a large pedigree afflicted with a particular genetic illness also has the 5-kb restriction fragment. This is strongly suggestive of the linkage of the unknown mutant allele to the chromosomal segment that contains this particular RFLP (Figure 3–5). This example illustrates the importance of heterozygosity in linkage analysis because if every ill member of the pedigree is homozygous (both copies of a particular gene or marker on a pair of homologous chromosomes are exactly alike) for this particular marker, no distinction can be made between the chromosome that contains the normal allele and the one that contains the mutant allele. To establish linkage to this particular region, an investigator would be obliged to search for additional RFLP markers that are heterozygous in the pedigree being analyzed.

A more typical experimental scenario takes place when an investigator has no prior information concerning the chromosomal location of an unknown mutant allele responsible for a particular genetic illness. In this example, DNA extracted from a number of members of an informative pedigree are subjected to a random search involving hundreds of polymorphic markers derived from virtually every chromosome. Statistical analysis is performed to determine whether linkage exists between the illness and one particular chromosome-specific RFLP. This procedure is extremely labor intensive and may engage a moderately sized laboratory for several years. Once a reliable marker is found, investigators usually attempt to identify additional markers in the region to further narrow the search for the gene of interest to smaller and smaller chromosomal segments. Identifying the chromosomal region that contains a gene of interest by linkage

Basic Principles in Linkage Analysis   63

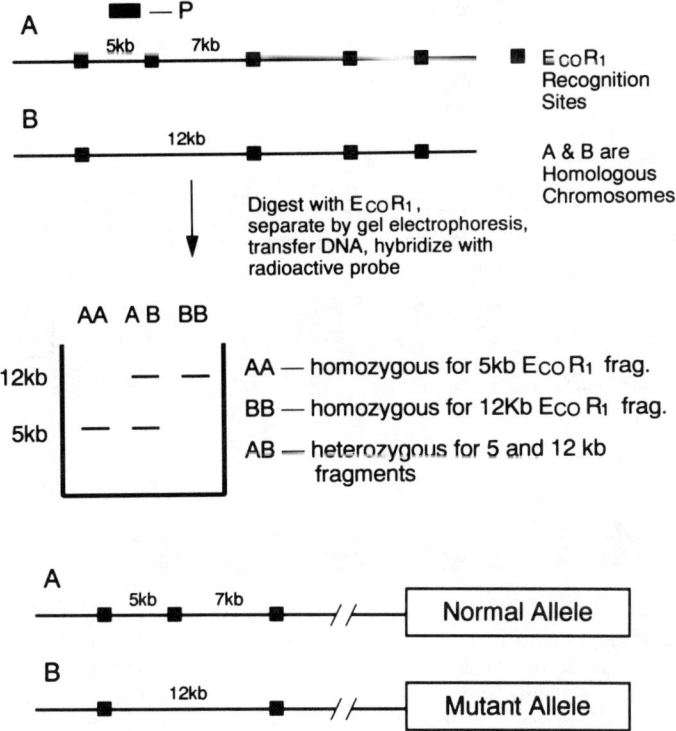

Figure 3–4. RFLP linkage analysis. Two homologous chromosomes (A and B) are shown that are virtually identical except that there is a loss of an *EcoRI* restriction endonuclease recognition signal on chromosome B (note that the homologous pair represents both copies of the same chromosome, such as chromosome 11). Using a radiolabeled probe (P) that is complementary to this region, different DNA bands will be generated. It should be noted that the probe does not have to span the entire region in order to detect the 5-and 12-kb fragments. In RFLP linkage analysis, a normal and a mutant allele are linked to chromosomes that contain one or the other restriction polymorphism (bottom of figure). In this example, individuals who inherit the mutant allele coinherit the 12-kb fragment and normal individuals the 5-kb fragment. The RFLP and the genes of interest are likely to be rather far apart (broken line). Although recombination is not shown on this figure, it should be apparent that if recombination such as that seen in Figure 3–3(C) should occur between the alleles of interest and the linked RFLP markers, some individuals will inherit a mutant allele with the 5-kb fragment rather than the 12-kb fragment.

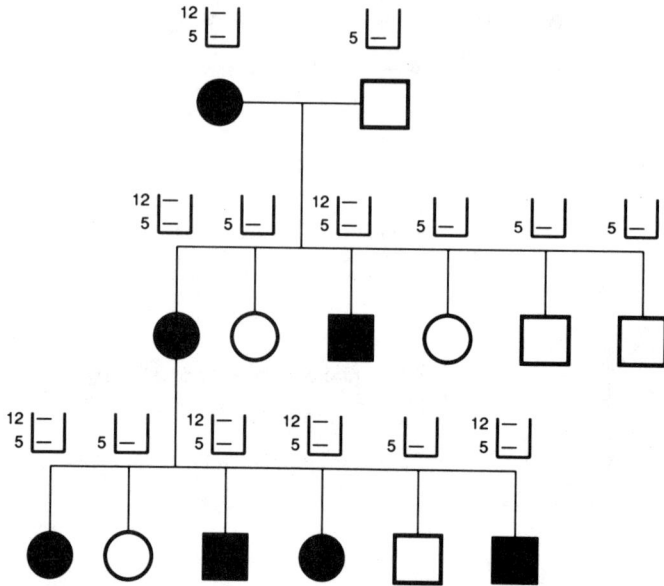

Figure 3–5. RFLP analysis in a pedigree. Affected individuals are depicted by the solid circles and squares. On the top of each member of the pedigree is a DNA gel electrophoresis pattern showing the RFLP bands derived from Figure 3–4. In this three-generation family, every individual who has the mutant phenotype has also inherited the 12-kb band, a finding that more likely is due to linkage of the mutant allele to the RFLP than to chance (statistical analysis would be performed to confirm this).

analysis restricts the search for an unknown gene from anywhere in the genome to a DNA segment that may contain only 5–10 million nucleotides, a 500-fold purification. Thus, in an unfolded DNA molecule that is 3 feet long, a gene of interest theoretically could be localized to a DNA fragment that is $1/14$ of an inch. Although this would constitute an important first step, a DNA fragment this size may still contain 100–200 different genes and much additional work would be required to isolate the hidden single gene of interest.

To help isolate the gene of interest, it is important that RFLP markers on both sides of the putative gene of interest, so-called flanking markers, be identified. In the absence of flanking markers, it is difficult for investigators to determine whether to "walk" across the DNA toward the gene of interest by moving, on a molecular level, to the right or to the left. Although it is beyond the scope of this chapter to discuss the cloning strategy in any great detail, suffice it to say that this, too, is labor intensive, and involves variations on the cloning strategies described earlier. Essentially, investigators "walk" or "jump" across the region, cloning and sequencing adjacent fragments until the gene of interest is found. The probability of finding a gene of interest is enhanced if it is expressed in a tissue-specific manner. For example, the manic-depressive vulnerability gene should be expressed in the brain. Therefore, fragments of DNA from the region under investigation could be examined for CNS expression.

With perseverance and luck, the target gene can be identified and the payoff can be monumental. In 1985, Tsui and colleagues identified an RFLP marker on chromosome 7 that was tightly linked to the development of cystic fibrosis, the most common autosomal recessive disorder in Caucasians (Tsui et al., 1985). Only four years later, following a well-orchestrated effort implemented by several large and well-established groups of investigators, the gene responsible for cystic fibrosis was identified (Rommens et al., 1989; Kerem et al., 1989).

Not every DNA linkage study results in the rapid identification of genes of interest. In 1983, a chromosome 4 RFLP marker was found to be linked to the development of Huntington's disease in a large Venezuelan family with a multigeneration history of the illness (Gusella et al., 1983). Compared with manic-depressive disorder, Huntington's disease is a simple genetic illness—autosomal dominance with 100% penetrance. Yet, despite a fairly intensive search, the gene responsible for this fascinating neuropsychiatric condition has not yet been cloned.

CANDIDATE GENE APPROACH

Because of the problems inherent in using random RFLP in studying manic-depressive disorder, an alternative approach is to analyze RFLPs in the region of specific candidate genes. A gene could be considered a candidate in manic-depressive disorder based on its role in regulating a biochemical or electrophysiological pathway thought to be involved in the etiology of mood disorders. For example, according to the catecholamine hypothesis, one would consider that the genes encoding regulators of adrenergic neurotransmission, such as the β-adrenergic receptors (β-AR), would be appropriate candidates

(Bunney & Davis, 1965). Rather than perform a large-scale RFLP search involving the entire genome, one can attempt to establish linkage using informative RFLPs located within the β-receptor gene locus. A study by Gershon and colleagues using this approach failed to demonstrate linkage to the β-AR gene in a pedigree with manic-depressive illness (Hoehe, Berrettini, & Gershon, 1989). Other sets of potential candidate genes under consideration include those encoding various components of the muscarinic cholinergic and serotonergic pathways, which are transmitter systems thought to be involved in the pathogenesis of mania and depression respectively (Janowsky, Risch, Parker, Huey, & Judd, 1980; Dilsaver, 1986; Van Pragg, 1979).

There are two major problems with the candidate gene approach. One is that it suffers from the same handicap as random RFLP linkage analysis with respect to diagnostic issues (see Chapter 2). Another problem is that the list of potential candidate genes is too extensive to be very useful. For example, if one believes in the cholinergic hypothesis of mania, then not only are the genes encoding muscarinic receptor subtypes potential candidates, but those encoding the transducing and target systems coupled to the muscarinic receptors also should be considered. Furthermore, a genetic defect leading to reduced cholinergic drive may not involve the muscarinic system directly, but could conceivably lie in an interacting pathway involving a completely different neurotransmitter system. In this scenario, literally hundreds of different candidate genes are possible.

CONCLUSION

There are no easy solutions to the problems associated with determining the genetic defects involved in manic-depressive disorder. Probably the most reasonable approach is to improve the diagnostic tools and the computer programs involved in analyzing multigenic conditions that exhibit variable penetrance, as discussed in detail in Chapters 2 and 5. Finding a reliable phenotypic marker to help distinguish between asymptomatic carriers of abnormal alleles and normal individuals would be enormously helpful. For example, abnormal eye tracking found in schizophrenics and well family members may be a biological trait-dependent marker in schizophrenia (Holzman et al., 1988). The search for informative pedigrees should also be a major priority. It is conceivable that extremely informative pedigrees exist that exhibit unequivocal diagnostic criteria and a single dominant genetic locus. Even if the gene or genes that underlie manic-depressive vulnerability in this hypothetical pedigree are a rare cause of illness, the discovery of the first vulnerability gene will undoubtedly provide information that will make the search for additional genes less difficult; we will have the molecular equivalent of the Rosetta Stone.

Improved DNA polymorphism maps will also increase the probability of finding genes of interest. Every year, human geneticists identify hundreds of new RFLP markers, resulting in more extensive maps of the genome. The earliest maps generated using RFLP markers were limited because some chromosomes were underrepresented. Like geographical maps, as more detail is added, the easier it is to find your way. The resolution of current maps is at a level of sophistication such that virtually any position in the genome can be placed within approximately 5 to 10 million bases of an RFLP marker. For some chromosomal regions, the map is even more saturated, with DNA polymorphisms marking these areas every one million base pairs. Supersaturated maps, combined with the mechanization of DNA probing strategies and computer analysis, will make the search for unknown genes more efficient.

Finally, the Human Genome Project will add a new dimension to the gene searches. The objectives of the project, which is fittingly directed by James Watson, are to map and eventually clone the entire human genome over the next few decades. Considering the information explosion occurring on so many fronts, it would not be surprising if at least one mutant allele responsible for the vulnerability to manic-depressive disorder were to be uncovered during the professional lives of many readers of this book.

REFERENCES

Berrettini, W. H., Cappellari, C. B., & Gershon, E. H. (1987). Beta-adrenergic receptor function in manic depressive illness. *Biological Psychiatry, 22,* 1439–1443.

Bishop, J. M. (1991). *Cell.* Elsevier.

Botstein, D., White, R. L., Skolnick, M., & Davis, R. W. (1980). Construction of a genetic linkage map in humans using restriction fragment length polymorphism. *American Journal of Human Genetics, 32,* 314–331.

Bunney, W. E., & Davis, J. (1965). Norepinephrine in depressive reactions. *Archives of General Psychiatry, 13,* 483–494.

Darnell, J., Lodish, H., & Baltimore, D. (1990). *Molecular cell biology.* New York: Scientific American Books.

Dilsaver, S. C. (1986). Cholinergic mechanisms in depression. *Brain Research Reviews, 11,* 285–316.

Gusella, J. F., Wexler, N. S., Conneally, P. M., Naylor, S., Anderson, M. A., Tanzi, R. E., Watkins, P. C., Ottina, K., Wallace, M. R., Sakaguchi, A. Y., Yound, A. B., Shoulson, I., Bonilla, E., & Martin, J. B. (1983). A polymorphic DNA marker genetically linked to Huntington's disease. *Nature, 306,* 234–238.

Hoehe, M. R., Berrettini, W. H., & Gershon, E. S. (1989). Adrenergic receptor genes and their role in manic-depressive illness. *Biological Psychiatry, 25,* 147A. Abstract presented at 43rd annual meeting of the Society of Biological Psychiatry.

Holzman, P. S., Kringlen, E., Mattheysse, S., Flanagan, S. D., Lipton, R. B., Cramer, G., Levin, S., Lange, K., & Levy, D. L. (1988). A single dominant gene can account for eye tracking dysfunctions and schizophrenia. *Archives of General Psychiatry, 45*(7), 641–647.

Janowsky, D. S., Risch, S. C., Parker, D., Huey, L. Y., & Judd, L. (1980). Increased vulnerability to cholinergic stimulation in affective disorder patients. *Psychopharmacology Bulletin, 16,* 29–31.

Kerem, B., Rommens, J. M., Buchanan, J. A., Markiewicz, D., Cox, T. K., Chakravarti, A., Buckwald, M., & Tsui, L.-C. (1989). Identification of the cystic fibrosis gene: Genetic analysis. *Science, 245,* 1073–1080.

Meselson, M., & Yuan, R. (1968). DNA restriction enzymes from *E. coli. Nature, 217,* 1110.

Monaro, A. P., Neve, R. L., Collett-Feener, C. A., Betelson, C. J., Kurnit, D. M., & Kunkel, L. M. (1986). Isolation of candidate cDNA for portions of Duchenne's muscular dystrophy gene. *Nature, 323,* 646–650.

Rommens, J. M., Iannuzzi, M. C., Keren, B., Drumm, M., Melmer, G., Dean, M., Rozmabel, R., Cole, G. L., Kennedy, D., Hidaka, N., Zsiga, M., Buchwald, M., Riordan, J. R., Tsui, L.-C., & Collins, F. S. (1989). Identification of the cystic fibrosis gene: Chromosome walking and jumping. *Science, 245,* 1059–1065.

Sambrook, J., Fritsch, E. F., & Maniatis, T. (1989). *Molecular cloning.* Cold Springs Harbor, NY: Cold Springs Harbor Laboratories Press.

Smith, H. (1979). Nucleotide sequence specificity of restriction enzymes. *Science, 205,* 455-462.

Tsui, L.-C., Buchwald, M., Barker, D., Braman, J. C., Knowlton, R., Schumm, J. W., Eiberg, H., Mohr, J., Kennedy, D., Plavsic, N., Zsiga, M., Markiewicz, D., Akots, G., Brown, V., Helms, C., Gravius, T., Parker, C., Rediker, K., & Donis-Keller, H. (1985). Cystic fibrosis locus defined by a genetically linked polymorphic DNA marker. *Science, 230,* 1054-1057.

Van Pragg, H. M. (1979). Central serotonin: Its relation to depression vulnerability and depressive prophylaxis. In J. Obiols, C. Balluus, E. Gonzales Manclus, & J. Pujol (Eds.), *Biological psychiatry today.* New York: Elsevier.

Watson, J. D., & Crick, F. H. C. (1953). Molecular structure of nucleic acids: A structure for deoxyribonucleic acid. *Nature, 171,* 737.

4

An Epidemiologic and Genetic Study of Affective Disorders among the Old Order Amish

JANICE A. EGELAND

A scientific account of the Amish Study accomplishes several objectives. It provides an overview of the genetic hypotheses, methods, and results for a research investigation that now spans a 16-year period, and yet remains contemporary in its aims and focus. It also illustrates the basic genetic research strategy during the period of the 1970s through the 1990s, a time that has brought revolutionary changes in the procedures and prospects for research in psychiatric genetics, and, indeed for all of medical genetics.

The significance of this period lies in the fact that we have moved from an era in which one could speak only in statistical terms about the probability of an illness's being genetic (family, twin, and adoption studies) through a period of traditional linkage and segregation studies (statistical programs), and into a molecular phase of linkage study. Although the basic methodology has remained the same, the potential is inherent in the newer recombinant DNA techniques. Results now eclipse mere mathematical statements. The individual DNA variations of well and ill individuals are visible portraits that may help to draft the hereditary blueprint of these common and devastating disorders.

With the availability of a linkage map, there now exists the promise of identifying genetic markers linked to the illness and eventually determining the location of a specific gene or genes crucial for elucidating the biochemical pathways in the brain that are associated with the cyclic illness known as manic-depressive disorder. Once there is a better understanding of the pathogenesis of this devastating illness, it should be possible to develop much more effective treatments with fewer side effects.

Just as this illness is cyclic in nature, so is the evolutionary process of research that is developmental and pioneering by definition. Certainly, the Amish Study can claim its fair share of the excitement of discovery and the sobering realities of replication. This chapter discusses the role of the study in facilitating an interface between the "old" psychiatric genetics and the "new" molecular biology of mental disorders.

THE AMISH SETTING: REQUISITES FOR GENETIC STUDY

It is rare for a researcher to have access to an entire population to study the distribution and etiology of a common medical condition. When that population is a "deme" (a "closed" genetic and culturally homogeneous group), the investigator has a truly unique research opportunity. This accurately describes the study of the Amish community located in southeastern Pennsylvania, the oldest and one of the largest Old Order Amish settlements in the United States.

The investigator must incorporate ethnographic and epidemiologic methods in order to enter such a closed group and to maintain long-term rapport with the population under study. Selection must be made from among the many research possibilities to focus on those with the greatest scientific merit and least cultural intrusion. One must protect the group by limiting contact with the families and respecting cultural boundaries.

With regard to mental illness, there are some important features that enhanced the proposed research. The investigator already knew of the existence of large families that have manifested manic-depressive disorder over the generations. The rate of illness in the population mirrors that of other communities, and the clinical characteristics of patients are indistinguishable between Amish and non-Amish. It was assumed that the Amish would appreciate and understand the goals of the research. This would ensure willing participation because they recognize and are deeply concerned about the symptoms and terrible suffering of the mentally ill.

Alcoholism, substance abuse, sociopathy, and family dissolution are infrequent among the Amish, whereas in other populations, these behaviors or events have complicated the ascertainment and accurate diagnosis of affective disorders. Therefore, a purer presentation of symptoms and a more classical natural history of the illness were expected. Moreover, an agrarian-based community, with a strong work ethic and an intolerance of malingering, would not be tolerant of somatic or "masked" depressive states. People are expected to resolve their physical and emotional complaints and return to their usual active social roles. Since the culture encourages expressions of sadness and grief (weeping is common at church), and since both men and women were at home for the interview procedure, it was assumed that the ascertainment of mood (affective) disorders would be enhanced for both sexes.

In addition to these positive features for the study of affective disorders, a number of widely recognized factors that are important for the study of any genetically transmitted condition are present in this population. These include:

- A closed, "inbred" community (i.e., genetic isolate with fewer genes that might predispose to the illness).
- Multigenerational families with large sibships for linkage study.
- Confidence regarding the paternity of subjects (essential for genotyping).
- Limited "out-migration" and geographic mobility so that extended-family members are available for study.
- Excellent genealogical records to trace ancestry.
- A notable cultural uniformity that reduces sources of variability in behaviors and beliefs.
- The cohesiveness of family and community life that provides a rich resource of patient observation by multiple informants.

In short, the study population is self-defined and genetically circumscribed. The principal investigator had developed close personal ties among the Amish beginning in 1959.

The long-term objective of this study was to clarify the genetic status of major affective disorders, with a specific focus on bipolar, or manic-depressive, illness. The questions posed by the study include: (1) Is there evidence of a genetic predisposition to major affective disorders? (2) What is the mode of transmission? (3) Are there genetic markers linked to a locus predisposing to the illness? (4) Within the spectrum of affective disorders, are there homogeneous subtypes?

EPIDEMIOLOGIC BASIS OF THE AMISH STUDY

The Amish Study was formally initiated in 1976 with funding from the National Institute of Mental Health (NIMH). Field work began with an epidemiologic survey of the entire community to ascertain accurate demographic information about all households, segregated by "church districts." These districts represent arbitrary geographic areas encompassing 20 to 30 families, the number that are able to assemble for worship within a home. It was possible to begin the formal case ascertainment while collecting the demographic data. Two methods for patient case ascertainment were used: multiple community informants and the screening of all admissions to psychiatric facilities in the area.

Once cases were identified, two methods were employed for clinical documentation. One included the abstraction of all psychiatric records and the other used multiple structured psychiatric interviews with patients and persons close to the patients. This process of case documentation was the basis for the formal diagnostic evaluations using strict Research Diagnostic Criteria (RDC) by a panel of five clinicians (Spitzer, Endicott, & Robins, 1978). These diagnostic procedures and their reliability were previously described (Hostetter, Egeland, & Endicott, 1983; Egeland et al., 1990).

It should be underscored that the *reliability* of diagnoses and the capacity for continuous follow-up of all family members are key elements in any genetic study; this is especially true for linkage studies.

The importance of the diagnostic effort supersedes all else and ideally should precede initiation of the blood-collection phase of a linkage study. A rush to collect blood samples prior to proper diagnostic evaluation of an extended family has been a flaw in many studies. After the fact, one commonly discovers problems of assortative mating, comorbidity, lack of cooperation by key subjects, and lack of consensus in diagnoses.

It has been the policy of the Amish Study investigators to perform systematic structured psychiatric interviews (and hospital record reviews) for all candidates for genetic linkage study prior to drawing blood samples. These "linkage" cases are mixed with others from the general community survey work so that the diagnostic panel is blind to proband status, family membership, and positive versus negative family histories. This "blindness" minimizes a bias toward the diagnosis of affective disorders within the sample of bipolar pedigrees under linkage study.

By 1980, we reported on the ascertainment of 112 "actively ill" patient cases; 71% had a major affective disorder according to the RDC (Egeland & Hostetter, 1983). A 1986 report listed 62%, or 107 of 173 patients, as actively ill with major affective disorders (Egeland, 1986). The latest diagnostic breakdown for active cases through the past 15 years is given in Table 4–1. Of 221 individuals, 138 (62.4%) were diagnosed with a bipolar or unipolar disorder.

Throughout the time frame of the Amish Study, the proportion of major depressive to bipolar illness has remained close to a 1:1 ratio: 1980, 41 unipolar compared with 38 bipolar or 52% compared with 48%; 1985, 56 unipolar compared with 51 bipolar or 52% compared with 48%; 1990, 69 unipolar compared with 69 bipolar or 50% of both forms of the illness. An early report based on the ascertainment of bipolar illness from the Amish Study recorded a 1:1 ratio of bipolar to unipolar disorder. This remarkable observation was referred to as the "iceberg of affective disorders" (Egeland, 1983). Previous studies, often based on institutional statistics, have reported a much higher (even 10:1) unipolar-to-bipolar ratio.

Although the majority of extant studies report a unipolar-to-bipolar ratio of 4:1, some investigations have found ratios of major depressive and manic-depressive cases closer to 1:1. For example, Bazzoui (1970)

TABLE 4-1
RDC Diagnoses of Amish Study
Active Cases: 1976-1990

RDC Diagnoses	Number	Percent
Bipolar I and II disorder	63	28.5
Other bipolar (atypical/chronic)	6	2.7
Unipolar major depression	69	31.2
Minor depressive disorder	22	9.9
Schizoaffective disorder	16	7.2
Schizophrenia	5	2.3
Atypical psychosis	2	0.9
Paranoid disorder	3	1.4
Obsessive-compulsive disorder	4	1.8
Psychosexual disorder	5	2.3
Generalized anxiety disorder	4	1.8
Anorexia	3	1.4
Cyclothymic disorder	2	0.9
Personality disorders	14	6.3
Other	3	1.4
TOTAL	221	100.0%

reported that 44% of all affective disorders were bipolar; Gershon and Liebowitz (1975) found 45% of the cases were bipolar in their Jerusalem study; and Angst (1978) and colleagues cited a 1:1 ratio for affectively ill patients who were followed over a 16-year period.

This point is emphasized to underscore the importance of mapping the terrain for bipolar II disorder, characterized by a pattern of hypomania and depression. Patients are deprived of vital treatment modalities because bipolar illness generally, and bipolar II in particular, has been widely under- or misdiagnosed. Additionally, researchers lose valuable opportunities to study genetic variants in the spectrum of affective disorders. For genetic linkage analyses, it may be more strategic to have ascertained all forms of bipolar disorder for incorporation into the analyses than to include all cases of major depression, such as those with single episodes or late onset.

With respect to sex ratios, we have found that there are no significant differences in the rates of bipolar and unipolar disorders between males and females in the Amish population. Among the 138 cases of bipolar and unipolar disorder shown in Table 4-1, there were 70 males and 68 females. (Note: There are equal numbers of males and females at each five-year period for the Amish population as a whole.) The increase in the number of males who were bipolar (40 male and 29 female) and the reverse for unipolar depression (39 female and 30 male) are not statistically significant, but are in the direction widely cited in the literature. Furthermore, it has been observed that morbid risk analyses when examined according to sex of proband and sex of first-degree relatives yield no significant differences (Pauls, Morton, & Egeland, 1992). Therefore, the bipolar and unipolar forms of affective disorder appear to have a symmetrical distribution in the Amish community.

CONVENTIONAL LINKAGE REVISITED

A genetic linkage study using conventional blood markers was formally initiated after the establishment of a sample of 32 bipolar subjects and the completion of a diagnostic assessment of their 303 first-degree and 565 second-degree relatives. The selection of five bipolar pedigrees from this original sample was based on a consideration of pedigree structure and size and the segregation of major affective disorders. These five pedigrees were ideal candidates and thought to be potentially informative for linkage. The first blood samples were drawn in 1979 when typing of the conventional blood markers began.

At this juncture, it might be helpful to describe a strategy built into the Amish Study, namely, that of making midcourse corrections and seeking options to maximize the potential of any given effort. The initial research goal was to replicate earlier reported findings of a positive linkage between affective illness and markers on the X chromosome: deutan and protan color blindness and the Xg blood group marker loci. The singular intent was to test this X-linkage hypothesis. It was decided, however, that in drawing blood samples from these families, all possible blood markers should be typed in order to test autosomal hypotheses as well. Consequently, a total of 94 family members were examined for color blindness, typed for the Xg blood group markers, and simultaneously typed for 42 red blood cell and related markers in 17 antigen systems. Finally, 59 individuals in two additional large bipolar pedigrees (already typed for the above) were also screened for the human leukocyte antigen (HLA) system, including BF and GLO.

Research reports of a positive linkage between HLA markers and depression had influenced the expansion of our typing program. The phase of testing conventional blood markers continued through 1982.

Results from the various linkage analyses using the conventional blood markers were published in a single report (Kidd et al., 1984). The red cell Xg locus was uninformative in the Amish Study, as is the case for most published studies on non-Amish pedigrees. Our pedigree data did not support X linkage; the magnitudes of the most negative lod (Log_{10} [odds ratio]) scores exceeded those of the most positive, using a variety of diagnostic schemes with LIPED. Typed markers on ABO, COMT, Rh, Duffy, Kidd, MNSs, P_1, Lewis, Yk^a, Cs^a, McC^a, and KN^a were tested and analyses done assuming autosomal inheritance. There was some evidence that suggested linkage to markers ABO, MNSs, YK^a, and Kn^a. However, strong linkage of affective disorders to these markers was not supported. Finally, the evidence was against close linkage to chromosome 6 HLA markers.

In short, we tested a number of uninformative and/or negative markers but did not locate any potential genetic marker for major affective disorders. These kinds of "negative" findings can dampen the enthusiasm of a researcher—but they should not. Science is the orderly "ruling out" of hypotheses that are alternative to the "null," and one should always be prepared for the next avenue of exploration. The dead ends in science exist for those who forget to turn a corner. For us, this was a shift in direction away from the use of conventional blood markers to the new DNA techniques applied to psychiatric linkage study.

PARALLEL GENETIC AVENUES: INHERITANCE PATTERNS

Recall that one of the stated aims of the Amish Study was to seek evidence for the mode of transmission of bipolar illness, as reflected in *segregation analyses*. These analyses have been conducted at several points in the Amish Study, first with a sample of 32 bipolar pedigrees and at present with an expanded sample numbering 38 bipolar families. Results from the analyses of the initial sample of 32 pedigrees indicated that the mode of transmission for affective disorders among the Old Order Amish was consistent with an autosomal dominant inheritance (D. L. Pauls, personal communication). Hypotheses of "no genetic transmission" of polygenic and recessive modes of inheritance could be rejected at high levels of statistical confidence. (Note: These initial analyses were done without incorporating information about inbreeding in this population. While it is unlikely that including information on consanguinity will alter the results cited here, we are currently reanalyzing the expanded sample including this information.)

For our sample of 32 bipolar pedigrees, the model of autosomal dominance was shown to have a moderately high penetrance of 63%. An even higher penetrance of 85% was calculated for bipolar pedigree, 110 being used for linkage study. The gene frequency for the susceptibility allele was estimated to be 0.021 (Egeland et al., 1987). The importance of performing segregation analyses parallel to linkage analyses is that they serve to define the variables (penetrance estimates, gene frequency, etc.) needed to conduct the linkage analyses.

The diagnostic scheme showing the best "goodness-of-fit" in support of the dominant gene model includes the following diagnoses: bipolar I, bipolar II, schizoaffective disorder (manic and depressed subtypes), atypical bipolar disorder, and major depressive disorder. These particular disorders appear to share a common genetic diathesis. The inclusion of minor depressive disorder and other milder conditions in the diagnostic scheme weakened the evidence for single gene transmission and do not appear to be part of the same genetic diathesis. This does not preclude the possibility that some subjects with these conditions or other disorders within the affective spectrum may have a milder manifestation of the inherited illness. Further investigations are needed to examine these questions.

Segregation analyses that indicated that autosomal dominant inheritance was most consistent with the pattern of illness observed in the Amish bipolar pedigrees proved to be a major impetus to our linkage study. The recent analyses for the expanded sample of 42 families confirms a dominant gene in certain bipolar pedigrees. An exciting prospect for the future (discussed in Chapter 5) is the possibility of working with newer genetic models that should allow two or more trait loci (genes) to be examined simultaneously by linkage analyses.

A second and unique methodology built into the Amish Study relates to ascertaining the inheritance of manic-depressive illness by means of the Progenitor Trace Study. Questions that are central to this approach include: Is there proof of a single and/or multiple gene pathways for mental illness tracked over the generations? Can one trace the introduction of the putative bipolar gene into the Old Order Amish settlement?

All present-day Amish living in the Lancaster, PA area and related settlements descend from relatively few Swiss Brethren and German founders, numbering around 30 original couples. They migrated to southeastern Pennsylvania between 1730 and 1770. For over 30 years, this writer has been doing a genealogical study of this community and assembling extensive evidence of early mental disorders using court, hospital, state, and other records. With this information, it is possible to construct "pedigree profiles" for recurrent, serious psychiatric illness on a historical basis.

It has been of interest to me that the farther back one searches for evidence of psychiatric disorder, the more males predominate in the ascertainment. Likewise, if one looks at the psychiatric status of parents of all RDC-confirmed bipolar I cases to date (active or inactive), one finds only a few instances where the mother, rather than the father, was affected. (Note: In the entire sample, 55% = neither parent was diagnosable with a major affective disorder, 9% = only the mother was affected, and 29% = only the father was affected.) Almost without exception, the affected father had a bipolar form of the disorder (80% bipolar). Yet this phenomenon of "male bipolar" lineage must be viewed in context. Males with bipolar illness have been able to marry at a much higher rate than have females with the disorder.

In the sample of actively ill patients, about half of all bipolar women are married as compared with 74% of the bipolar men (87% of adult Amish marry). Historically, there appear to be even fewer instances where a woman with a serious bipolar illness was encouraged or permitted to undertake the responsibilities of marriage and motherhood. Those few who did marry undoubtedly showed few or no symptoms prior to marriage. Contrary to this bias, the man was expected to be married and was helped with any difficulty, including physical deformity, mental retardation, or psychiatric illness. Today, when a male teenager exhibits the signs and symptoms of acute mania, one still hears the comment that what he needs is a good "helpmate." Marriage

80   *Basic Methods, Current Directions, and Critical Research Issues*

with some stable young woman is encouraged. The opposite scenario is rare. The female bipolar is not as likely to be "predisposing" her young to bipolar affective disorder, either by virtue of her genetic endowment or her "maladaptive" parenting influences when sick.

Using both community informants and earlier court and psychiatric institution records, no serious mental disorder can be ascertained for most of the pioneer couples and their immediate descendants. This is equally true for contemporary families; the community rate for major affective disorders is not enhanced. However, there is an obvious clustering of psychopathology for selected family lines, documented as early as the first, second, and third generations. An example is given in Figure 4–1A, shown in summary form with deletion of sibships for the sake of brevity.

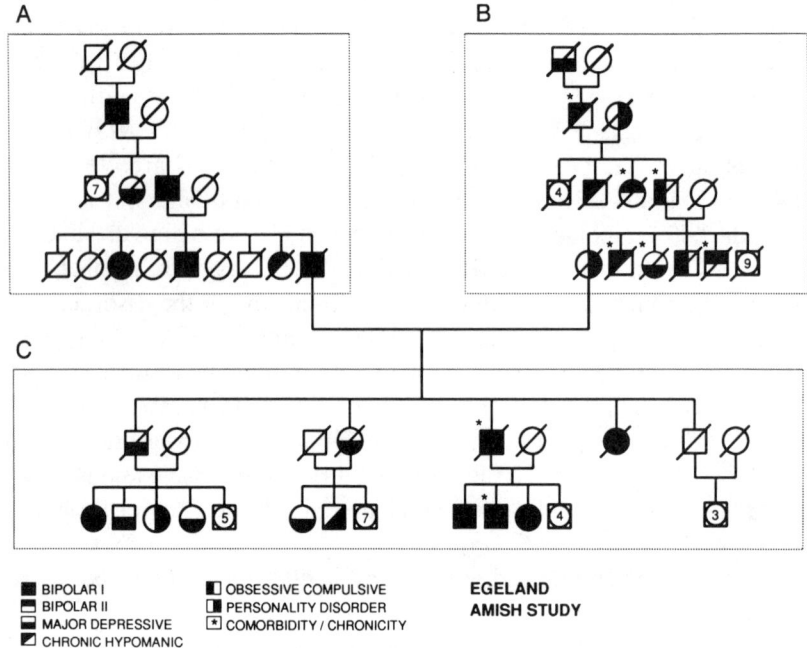

Figure 4–1.

Figure 4–1A indicates that bipolar I disorder is evident in each successive generation from the progenitor. This pedigree profile is very characteristic of many present-day bipolars, who trace directly along this historic pathway; there is a heavy loading for bipolar I and major depression and very little else. You do not see the comorbidity or the spectrum of illness as depicted in Figure 4–1B.

In contrast, Figure 4–1B illustrates a pioneer Amish family where the son (shown as generation I) was despondent and is said to have taken his life while in his 30s. Successive generations are found to have a variety of mental illnesses, including definite major depression and several cases of chronic hypomania. By generation III, there is one documented case of a bipolar II. No evidence of mania can be found in family or institutional records.

Figure 4–1C shows a marriage between these two family lines. It is at this point that bipolar I illness enters the family seen in Figure 4–1B. Prior to the marriage between the two generation IV individuals, a definite bipolar I pathway was ascending only to the one pioneer couple. By using this strategy for plotting the illness, it is now possible to reject as "carriers" most pioneer couples and to confirm the few progenitors who are candidates for transmission of this bipolar heritage.

Uncertainties attend this type of traditional hand-tracing of pedigree profiles. It is not sufficient to use these pedigree profiles as proof of the pathways for bipolar illness to particular pioneers. Significant differences in the progenitor traces for the sample of bipolar patients compared with a random control sample should be proved. This requires constructing a statistical program for use with the computer program that allows us to trace any given person back to all progenitors by all possible pathways.

Completion of the Progenitor Trace Study should yield data regarding the existence of one, or more than one, major gene predisposing to bipolar affective disorder in the Amish population. It could provide data on the genetic homogeneity of confirmed cases of major affective disorder. This might dictate a division of pedigrees and sibships for separate linkage analyses. In other words, it could sharpen the focus of genetic linkage analysis for homogeneous subtypes of the illness.

This is one of the most exciting parallel avenues traveled in the quest for answers to genetic questions about both the inheritance and homogeneity of subtypes of the illness.

GENETIC LINKAGE BY DNA METHODS

No DNA restriction fragment length polymorphisms (RFLPs) had been detected in humans at the time the Amish Study was funded in 1976. By 1979, when our first blood samples were drawn for typing of the conventional blood markers, polymorphism detection was still hampered by the lack of cloned probes at the DNA level. Only one DNA polymorphism was known to exist in humans (Kan & Dozy, 1978; Southern, 1978). Subsequently, the rate at which these DNA polymorphisms could be generated accelerated beyond all expectations. Molecular biology provided a new technology to be applied to genetic linkage studies. Researchers predicted that the mapping of the human genome could be accomplished within a decade. It was time to apply the DNA methods to the search for genetic markers linked to a psychiatric condition; bipolar disorder was clearly a candidate and the Amish Study undertook to initiate the effort.

In 1982, one large Amish bipolar pedigree was selected from the original sample of five. By 1983, the DNA was available on 51 subjects and the first molecular genetic study of bipolar disorder was launched. Many collaborators contributed to this original effort. The RFLPs studied at Yale, in Dr. K. Kidd's laboratory, made it possible to rule out a number of markers on different chromosomes (Kidd et al., 1987). Extensive mapping on the short arm of chromosome 11 by Dr. D. Gerhard took place at The Massachusetts Institute of Technology in Dr. D. Housman's laboratory. Linkage analyses suggested that a major locus might exist on chromosome 11, and these findings were reported as "provocative," but certainly not definitive (Gerhard et al., 1984).

In order to confirm or reject these preliminary findings, 30 additional blood samples were collected in 1984 from other close relatives in the same Amish family, pedigree 110. The total sample now consisted of 81 individuals; 19 had an RDC diagnosis of major affective disorders and 62 persons were considered unaffected. Genotypings were conducted blind to diagnoses. When the linkage analyses were completed, chromosome 11 markers were reported as being strongly linked to a locus predisposing to the illness (Egeland et al., 1987). This report received much scientific and public media attention.

The findings were robust. Genetic markers included insulin (INS) and the cellular oncogene Harvey-ras (HRAS), located on the short arm of chromosome 11p15. Lod scores were consistently over 3.0 using a wide range of parameters. (Note: A lod score of 3.0 or more gives odds of at least 1000 to 1 against this pattern occurring by chance alone.) When multipoint linkage analyses were conducted, using INS and HRAS marker loci simultaneously, the lod score was 4.9 (odds approaching 100,000 to 1).

This was the first scientific report on the localization of a gene conferring a predisposition to a common psychiatric condition using markers identified by means of recombinant DNA techniques. The attention drawn to the effort had a number of positive consequences. Coupled with other research reports in psychiatry, it provided the impetus to apply the DNA techniques to linkage study of psychiatric disorders and to foster increased funding for such studies.

Equally exciting was the extent to which the public began to learn about manic-depressive illness from the media and from books directed toward the general public (Papolos & Papolos, 1987). Patients and their families reported feeling less stigmatized and more likely to seek medical treatment for the condition. The timing of the Amish Study report corresponded to a plethora of articles on Alzheimer's disease, cystic fibrosis, familial cancer, and other conditions being examined in light of the new techniques of "reverse genetics."

REALITIES OF REPLICATION

Between 1979 (when only one DNA polymorphism was reported in humans) and 1983 (when over 200 RFLPs had been mapped), it seemed that we had passed from the Middle Ages to a modern era in human genetics. But everyone on the Amish Study research team knew at the time of the 1987 *Nature* article (Egeland et al., 1987) that the "highs" of discovery might be dampened by the realities of the long-term effort. We had already initiated a replication study.

There were a number of difficult problems to resolve, apart from a simple extension of our pedigree. First, there was the need for continuous follow-up of all subjects and this had to be done "blind" to genotype information. In any linkage study, a change in psychiatric status can impinge on the magnitude and direction of a lod score. We knew that continued emphasis on the reliability of diagnoses and a careful charting of variant or milder forms of the illness were important. Of course, diagnoses must be done blind to family relationships and genotypes. We realized it was probably best to define a number of diagnostic hierarchies and were working on that concept with the project's psychiatric board.

We acknowledged that it is an "art" as well as a science to read or interpret the DNA patterns on an autoradiograph. As with a controversial x-ray, it is necessary to establish reliability checks on these "molecular" measurements. Equally important was the realization of the necessity for appropriate statistical methods with the power and accuracy to test linkage and to understand the influence of varying the parameters. So the study was monitoring all critical levels of reliability: diagnoses, genotypes, and calculations.

By 1987, the Miami field staff had already expanded pedigree 110 from the original 81 subjects reported in *Nature* to include six new family members in a small left-hand extension and a larger, 31-member right-hand extension. The typing of chromosome 11 markers was begun in Dr. Gerhard's laboratory at Washington University. The fully expanded pedigree 110 numbered 120 subjects, 31 of whom had a diagnosis of one or more episodes of major affective disorder. This included two onsets for individuals previously unaffected in the core pedigree.

The cell collection for the Amish Study is unique in that it is available to the entire scientific community. Old Order Amish pedigree 110 was the first large reference pedigree for bipolar affective disorder to become part of the permanent cell repository at the Coriell Institute for Medical Research (CIMR) in Camden, NJ. Over 40 investigators have obtained some or all of the cell lines through the National Institute of General Medical Science (NIGMS) *Cell Repository Catalog.*

Sparked by the Amish Study findings, an NIMH group, headed by Dr. Steven Paul, director of Intramural Research (including Drs. J. Kelsoe, E. Ginns, and R. Long) had obtained the Amish cell lines and had examined tyrosine hydroxylase (on 11p15) as a candidate gene for bipolar affective disorder. In the process, they retyped the entire original sample, adding the new cell lines from the extensions. Dr. Paul proposed a collaborative effort, which resulted in the next major publication. It illustrated the several methodological steps outlined above and presented evidence that greatly diminished hopes of a linkage between a bipolar affective disorder gene locus and markers on chromosome 11p15 (Kelsoe et al., 1989).

Core Pedigree 110

The first fact to report is that a retyping of all individuals (with several discrepant typings resolved by further retyping) and a reanalysis using the original diagnoses produced results that replicated the 1987 report.

However, subsequent changes that involved the original core pedigree served to reduce the lod score to below 2.0. This overall reduction had three components. A 1.26 lod score reduction was due to a "single episode," late-onset "situational" depression. This raised the question of phenocopies—persons whose illness may be clinically indistinguishable but etiologically different. A second part of the lod score reduction was an even greater surprise because it was for a recent-onset bipolar I subject whose genotype was exactly that of other ill relatives in the original core pedigree. Yet the maximum lod score for INS was reduced by 0.76. At the time, this was especially difficult to understand. Recent simulation studies document that not all sibships within a pedigree structure are equally informative (Pauls & Egeland, 1990). Depending on the genotype for other subjects within these sibships who might still onset, the lod score could shift in either a more negative or a more positive direction.

A third source of reduction in the lod scores was brought about by updated genotypes for 10 individuals on whom only one of the two typings was available for the 1987 published findings. These were all unaffected subjects for whom the updated genotypes changed the maximum lod scores for both HRAS (decreased from 4.08 to 2.46) and INS (increased from 2.63 to 3.38 at θ = 0). Once these updated genotypes were factored into the analyses, along with the two new onsets, the lod score dropped below 2.0. This lowered lod score does not permit an actual exclusion of linkage to chromosome 11p15 markers for the core pedigree.

Extensions to Pedigree 110

The most sobering note was struck with the extremely *negative* lod scores for chromosome 11 markers typed in the new right extension made up of 31 subjects (four having bipolar I and three with major depression). When the extension was analyzed as a separate pedigree, the data revealed significantly negative lod scores for both INS and HRAS markers, sufficient to exclude at least 10 map units around INS and three map units around HRAS. Furthermore, when this new large extension was joined to the core as a single pedigree, the results remained negative. Multipoint analyses suggested that the whole region could be excluded on either side of INS and HRAS, representing some 10 million base pairs of DNA (Kelsoe et al., 1989).

Several explanations were proposed to address the fact that the 11p markers could not be excluded for the core pedigree itself where a small positive lod score that does not reach statistical significance still exists. (More onsets within the core could help to determine the direction of the earlier linkage report.) However, the original results could have been a false positive owing to such factors as sample size (n = 81) and sibship location of informative subjects.

A major explanation for the overall negative results in pedigree 110 core plus extensions could be that of genetic heterogeneity. Specifically, the right extension negative data could have been due to the introduction of a bipolar gene carried by a woman who married into the family.

Pedigree 210 as Another Major Extension

As a further step in replication, another large family, pedigree 210, was established for molecular study. Manifesting a six generation pattern for bipolar affective illness, it tied to pedigree 110 in the same structural manner as the previous large right extension. The 210 core consisted of 50 subjects, with 13 diagnosed as having major affective disorder. The chromosome 11p loci that were typed included HRAS, INS, TH, D11S12, HBBC, CALCA, FSH, and CAT. Results from both pairwise and multipoint analyses were uniformly and significantly negative for these markers (Pauls et al., 1991). The exclusion area encompassed approximately 68 map units on the short arm of chromosome 11. Hence, the linkage conclusions were consistent with those reviewed above.

MARATHON OF MARKERS

To meet this challenge, more cell lines have been added to the existing bipolar pedigrees, as summarized in Table 4–2. There are 231 cell lines for pedigrees 110 and 210 now available to those scientists involved in DNA study.

The diagnostic status of the subjects represented in Table 4–2 was as follows: 30 = bipolar I; 4 = bipolar II or atypical bipolar; 19 = major depressive disorder; 2 = schizoaffective disorder (bipolar or circular subtype); 11 = minor depressive disorder; 8 = other diagnoses considered unaffected for linkage purposes (atypical psychosis, personality disorder, anxiety disorder, etc.); 157 = no psychiatric disorder (unaffected).

Another large bipolar family was screened recently in preparation for further expansion of the Amish cell collection and 33 cell lines were transformed in 1991–92. Given the limited gene pool for the Amish genetic isolate, the efforts to detect linkage have naturally been expanded.

A variety of diagnostic hierarchies have been defined by the project's psychiatric board that have altered the stringency of the criteria used. For initial linkage analyses, individuals included as affected must have an RDC diagnosis of bipolar I disorder. Only with a second-step

TABLE 4–2
Evolution of Old Order Amish Affective Disorder Cell Collection at the National Cell Repository, Coriell Institute (Sample: 231)

Cell Lines	1982	1984	1986	1987	1988	1989	1990
Ped. 110/210	52	44	55	15	10	19	36

analysis and a "looser" definition of the illness are cases of bipolar II and recurrent, major depressive disorder added. Furthermore, we have adopted a conservative position of using only recurrent, major depressive disorder in order to control for possible phenocopies (false positives) represented by some single episodes of depression.

Continued simulation studies by Dr. D. Pauls will help in determining the structural features of the pedigrees with respect to informativeness and polymorphism. This will facilitate decisions regarding which branches or kinship lines should be joined and which should be separated from one another for the testing of linkage. Should more than one gene predispose to illness in these large families, separation of the pedigree into different lineages may help to locate a specific gene.

Through the Clinical Neuroscience Branch, Intramural Research Program (IRP) of the NIMH, a systematic screening of the genome was initiated. More than 350 markers have been typed for over 200 individuals in pedigrees 110–210. These markers are spaced at approximately 15 centimorgans (or 15 million base pairs) apart. Linkage analyses are being performed using several diagnostic hierarchies, as well as different gene susceptibility and inheritance models. To date, no lod scores greater than 3.0 have been obtained. We continue to accumulate data from a large number of additional, highly informative markers along with continuous up-dating of the diagnostic status for both affected and normal subjects. This will help to saturate the map and make chromosomal regions more informative for linkage analyses. In addition to this systematic mapping, other approaches such as identification of candidate genes and screening for the presence of expanded Trinucleotide repeats are being pursued.

Dr. Ginns, who directs the IRP-NIMH genome collaboration with the Amish Study, believes that "well-documented, large pedigrees like those found in the Old Order Amish provide rare and invaluable opportunities for us to open windows that will reveal the genetic basis of manic-depressive illness" (Ginns et al., 1991). At a meeting of the American College of Neuropsychopharmacology, Dr. S. Paul remarked that for our collaborative team the hard work has now started. Our endeavor was described as "more like running a marathon than a 100-yard dash." It has become a marathon of genetic markers. We are prepared for a demanding race on an unknown course that may take years

REFERENCES

Angst, J. (1978). The course of affective disorders: II. Typology of bipolar manic-depressive illness. *Archives of Psychiatry and Neurological Sciences, 226,* 65–73.

Bazzoui, W. (1970). Affective disorder in Iraq. *British Journal of Psychiatry, 117,* 195.

Egeland, J. A. (1983). Bipolarity: The iceberg of affective disorders? *Comprehensive Psychiatry, 24* (4), 337–344.

Egeland, J. A. (1986). Cultural factors and social stigma for manic-depression: The Amish Study. *American Journal of Social Psychiatry, 6,* 279–286.

Egeland, J. A., Gerhard, D. S., Pauls, D. L., Sussex, J. N., Kidd, K. K., Allen, C. R., Hostetter, A. M., & Housman, D. E. (1987). Bipolar affective disorders linked to DNA markers on chromosome 11. *Nature, 325,* 783–787.

Egeland, J. A., & Hostetter, A. M. (1983). Amish Study I: Affective disorders among the Amish, 1976–1980. *American Journal of Psychiatry, 140,* 56–61.

Egeland, J. A., Sussex, J. N., Endicott, J., Hostetter, A. M., Offord, D. R., Schwab, J. J., Allen, C. R., & Pauls, D. L. (1990). The impact of diagnoses on genetic linkage study for bipolar affective disorders among the Amish. *Psychiatric Genetics, 1,* 5–18.

Gerhard, D. S., Egeland, J. A., Pauls, D. L, Kidd, J. R., Kramer, P. L., Housman, D. E., & Kidd, K. K. (1984). Is a gene for affective disorder located on the short arm of chromosome 11? *American Journal of Human Genetics, 36,* 3S.

Gershon, E. S., & Liebowitz, J. H. (1975). Sociocultural and demographic correlates of affective disorders in Jerusalem. *Journal of Psychiatric Research, 12,* 37–50.

Ginns, E. I., Keith, T., Egeland, J. A., Falls, K., Allen, C., Long, R. T., Phipps, P., Gravius, T., Olsson, K., Bailey, J., Pauls, D. L., & Paul, S. M. (1991). Update on the search for DNA markers linked to manic-depressive illness in the core and extensions of Old Order Amish pedigree 110. *Psychiatric Genetics, 2* (1), S6/1.

Hostetter, A. M., Egeland, J. A., & Endicott, J. (1983). Amish Study II: Consensus diagnoses and reliability results. *American Journal of Psychiatry, 140,* 62–66.

Kan, Y. W., & Dozy, A. M. (1978). Polymorphism of DNA sequence adjacent to human beta-globin structure gene: Relationship to sickle mutation. *Proceedings of the National Academy of Sciences (USA), 75,* 5631–5635.

Kelsoe, J. R., Ginns, E. I., Egeland, J. A., Gerhard, D. S., Goldstein, A. M., Bale, S. J., Pauls, D. L., Long, R. T., Kidd, K. K., Conte, G., Housman, D. E., & Paul, S. M. (1989). Re-evaluation of the linkage relationship between chromosome 11p loci and the gene for bipolar affective disorder in the Old Order Amish. *Nature, 342,* 238–243.

Kidd, K. K., Egeland, J. A., Molthan, L., Pauls, D. L., Kruger, S. D., & Messner, K. H. (1984). Amish Study IV: Genetic linkage study of pedigrees of bipolar probands. *American Journal of Psychiatry, 141,* 1042–1048.

Kidd, J. R., Egeland, J. A., Pakstis, A. J., Castiglione, C. M., Pletcher, B. A., Morton, L. A., & Kidd, K. K. (1987). Searching for a major genetic locus for affective disorder in the Old Order Amish. *Journal of Psychiatric Research, 21,* 577–580.

Papolos, D. F., & Papolos, J. (1992). *Overcoming depression.* New York: HarperCollins.

Pauls, D. L., & Egeland, J. A. (1990). A simulation study using an Old Order Amish pedigree: The effect of changes in diagnosis on the evidence for genetic linkage. *Proceedings, 29th Annual Meeting of the American College of Neuropsychopharmacology,* San Juan, Puerto Rico.

Pauls, D. L., Gerhard, D. S., Lacy, L. G., Hostetter, A. M., Allen, C. R., Bland, S. D., LaBuda, M. C., & Egeland, J. A. (1991). Linkage of bipolar affective disorders to markers on chromosome 11p is excluded in a second lateral extension of Amish pedigree 110. *Genomics, 11,* 730–736.

Pauls, D. L., Morton, L. A., & Egeland, J. A. (1992). Risks of affective illness among first degree relatives of bipolar I Old Order Amish probands. *Archives of General Psychiatry, 49,* 703–708.

Southern, E. M. (1978). Detection of specific sequences among DNA fragments separated by gel electrophoresis. *Journal of Molecular Biology, 98,* 503–517.

Spitzer, R., Endicott, J., & Robins, E. (1978). Research diagnostic criteria: Rationale and reliability. *Archives of General Psychiatry, 35,* 773–782.

5

Genetic Linkage Studies in Psychiatry
Strengths and Weaknesses

DAVID L. PAULS

Genetic linkage is a powerful methodology to help elucidate the underlying genetic mechanisms for inherited disorders. As discussed in Chapters 2, 3, and 4, this method has also been proposed to help us understand the genetics of psychiatric disorders. The purpose of this chapter is to give a brief overview of the methodology and to provide examples that illustrate some of the strengths and weaknesses of this method when applied to complex disorders.

Genetic linkage is defined as the violation of Mendel's law of independent assortment. That law states that the alleles (i.e., different forms of a gene) at two chromosomal locations (i.e., two loci) will assort independently and be transmitted to offspring in random combinations. For example, if an individual has genotype A_1A_2 at locus A and genotype B_1B_2 at locus B and the loci are not linked to each other, then the alleles at locus A and locus B will assort independently and four different types of gametes (A_1B_1, A_1B_2, A_2B_1, A_2B_2) will be produced in equal frequencies.

Nonindependent assortment occurs when genetic loci are positioned near each other on the same chromosome. When two genes are close together, specific combinations of alleles will be transmitted together (i.e., cosegregate) within families. Continuing with the example, if

---

Supported by National Institute of Mental Health Research Scientist Development Award MH-00508.

locus A is close to locus B on some chromosome, an individual will again produce four types of gametes, but now the gametes will not be in equal frequencies. The most common types of gametes will be those that represent the combination of alleles that occurred in each parent (i.e., the parental phase). The less frequent types of gametes will be the result of recombination.*

To illustrate phase, assume that a parent has allele A_1 on the same chromosome as allele B_2. Assume also that this parent is heterozygous for loci A and B. It follows, then, that the homologous chromosome in this parent will carry alleles A_2 and B_1. Thus A_1B_2 and A_2B_1 are the parental phases for this individual. If A and B are linked, these parental combinations of alleles will cosegregate in the offspring of this individual. When illnesses of unknown etiology are being studied, cosegregation within families of an allele at a known genetic locus (i.e., a marker locus) and an illness is taken as evidence that genetic linkage exists between an underlying gene that confers susceptibility for the disease and the marker locus.

The expectation that genetic linkage will be useful for the study of psychiatric conditions is reasonable given the success of this approach in delineating genetic loci for a variety of inherited neurological and metabolic diseases (c.f., Huntington's disease, cystic fibrosis, familial Alzheimer's disease, muscular dystrophy, fragile X mental retardation). A few years ago, there was considerable optimism that this approach would be useful in the study of psychiatric illnesses when several groups reported linkage of bipolar affective disorders and schizophrenia to different regions of the genome (Baron et al., 1987; Egeland et al., 1987; Mendlewicz et al., 1987; Sherrington et al., 1988). Unfortunately, it has not been possible to replicate these findings in independent samples of families (Detera-Wadleigh et al., 1987, 1989; Hodgkinson et al., 1987; Kennedy et al., 1988; St. Clair et al., 1989; Pauls et al., 1991). The inability to replicate these findings has

---

* During meiosis, homologous chromosomes synapse prior to the first meiotic division. During synapse, chromosomes can exchange parts through a process called crossing over. When a crossover occurs between two linked loci, there will be a new combination of alleles that is different from the parental combinations. These new combinations are referred to as recombinations. The frequency of recombinations between two genetic loci is a function of the distance between them. The closer loci are to each other, the less likely it is that there will be a crossover/recombination between them.

been disappointing and has caused some investigators to question whether genetic linkage can be used successfully in the study of complex psychiatric disorders.

METHODS FOR THE DETECTION OF GENETIC LINKAGE

While these failures to replicate have dampened the initial enthusiasm for genetic linkage studies in psychiatry, the expectation that linkage studies will be useful in the elucidation of genetic factors important for the expression of psychiatric illness is still reasonable. The linkage-study approach has long been recognized as a powerful method for the identification of underlying genetic factors responsible for the manifestation of, or increased susceptibility for, specific disorders. Two approaches to linkage analyses have been developed: (1) the sib-pair method (Penrose, 1953; Suarez, Rice, & Reich, 1978), and (2) the family pedigree method (Morton, 1956). The sib-pair method is a model-free procedure (i.e., does not require any assumptions about the genetic mechanisms involved in the disease), whereas the family pedigree method requires that the mode of inheritance of the trait under study be specified. Since the mode of inheritance of any psychiatric disorder is not well understood, the sib-pair approach would seem to be the method of choice. However, sib-pair analyses are statistically less powerful than family pedigree analyses and do not allow the estimation of the recombination fraction and the strength of the linkage.* Nevertheless, the sib-pair approach can provide important preliminary evidence for linkage that can form the basis for more powerful techniques. For a more complete discussion of the sib-pair and other similar approaches, see Ott (1991).

---

* The strength of linkage is measured as the recombination fraction between a marker locus and the trait locus. The recombination fraction (θ) is a measure of the genetic distance between two loci and is expressed as the frequency of recombination observed in offspring between parental combinations of the alleles at the loci being examined. The closer two loci are to each other, the less likely it is that there will be a crossover or recombinant event between them. Thus θ can be used as a measure of genetic distance. The values of range from 0.0 (there is no recombination, the loci are right next to each other) to 0.5 (the loci are so far apart, or on separate chromosome, that random recombination occurs).

Initial linkage studies in human genetics involved known inherited disorders with complete penetrance.* Since the goal of these early studies was to estimate the recombination fraction, the family pedigree approach became the more widely used analytic method to test for linkage between an illness and a marker locus. It became even more widely used after the development of a computer program (LIPED) to facilitate the analysis of data from large families (Ott, 1976). The applicability of this approach to complex disorders was enhanced when LIPED was modified to allow for the incorporation of age- and sex-specific penetrance (Hodge, Morton, Tideman, Kidd, & Spence, 1979).

The family pedigree method involves the comparison of likelihoods[†] for specific genetic linkage hypotheses. First, the likelihood of observing a specific pattern of markers in a pedigree is calculated assuming the null hypothesis of no genetic linkage to be true. That is, the likelihood of observing the distribution of the disease and a set of marker genotypes is calculated assuming independent assortment of the disease and marker alleles. Next, the likelihoods of observing the pattern of disease and marker alleles for each of several alternative hypotheses of linkage are calculated and compared with the likelihood of the null hypothesis by means of an "odds ratio." The odds ratio consists of the likelihood of an alternative hypothesis divided by the likelihood of the null hypothesis. An odds ratio of greater than 1000 to 1 is taken as evidence for linkage, whereas an odds ratio of less than 1 in 100 is taken as evidence against linkage. For ease of comparison, the base 10 logarithm of the odds ratio is reported. In linkage analyses, these so-called "lod" scores ($\log_{10}$ [odds ratio]) are calculated for various hypotheses of linkage.

---

* Penetrance is defined as the probability that a specific genotype (i.e., the combination of alleles that a particular individual is carrying at a specific locus) will result in a specific phenotype. For example, a penetrance of 0.8 for genotype AA means that 80% of the time, an individual with genotype AA will exhibit the phenotype of interest. Alternatively, 20% of the time, an individual with genotype AA will not exhibit the phenotype. Complete penetrance refers to the situation in which the probability that a specific genotype will be expressed as a specific phenotype is 1.0.

† Likelihoods can be thought of as probabilities, although they are not exactly the same. Probabilities estimate the chance of observing data assuming a specific hypothesis to be true. Likelihoods estimate the chance that a hypothesis is true given the observed data. The actual calculations are essentially the same.

The alternative hypotheses of linkage are specified by different values of the recombination fraction. That is, the alternative hypotheses propose that (1) linkage is so close that no recombinations have occurred (i.e., $\theta = 0.0$); (2) linkage is tight, but a one-recombination event has occurred in 100 meioses ($\theta = 0.01$); (3) linkage is quite close, but relatively more recombinations have occurred ($\theta = 0.05$); and so on for increments of $\theta = 0.05$ until $\theta = 0.45$. The null hypothesis specifies that $\theta = 0.50$. A lod score greater than 3.0 ($\log_{10}$ [1000/1]) is taken as evidence for linkage and a lod score of less than -2.0 ($\log_{10}$ [1/100]) is taken as evidence against linkage. For a thorough discussion of linkage analysis, the reader is referred to the excellent book by Jurg Ott (1991).

To illustrate how lod scores are calculated, consider the family in Figure 5–1. An autosomal dominant disorder is segregating in this family. For the purposes of this example, assume that all affected individuals are heterozygotes. In order to calculate the likelihood of a

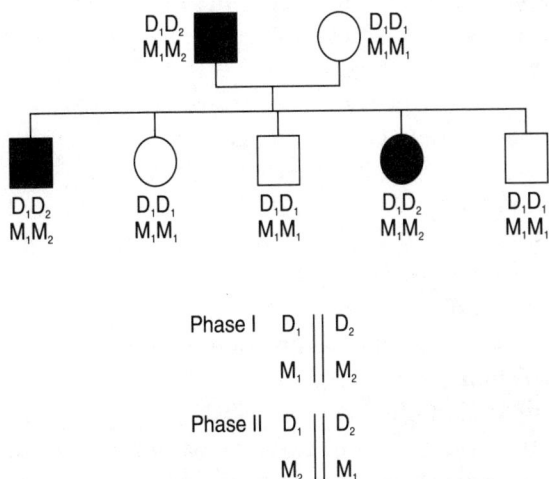

Figure 5–1. Pedigree of a family segregating an autosomal dominant trait. All affected individuals are assumed to be heterozygous. D_2 is the allele conferring susceptibility for the trait. D_1 is the normal allele at the D locus. M_1 and M_2 are the alleles of the marker locus. (*Note:* For any psychiatric illness, the D genotypes are assumed since it is not possible to type individuals for disease loci. Linkage analyses are undertaken to provide evidence that such a locus exists.)

particular family, it would be helpful to know the phase of each parent. Unfortunately, because it is not possible to type individuals for their disease alleles, it is not possible to determine the phase of the parents in this kindred directly. However, since the unaffected parent (I-2) can be assumed to be homozygous for the nonsusceptibility allele at the disease locus and is homozygous for the marker, the phase is known for that individual (i.e., D_1 is on the same chromosome as M_1).

Phase cannot be completely determined for the affected parent, but it is possible to narrow the possibilities. Because it is assumed that all affected individuals are heterozygous at the disease locus and it is known that this person is heterozygous at the marker locus, it follows that he is heterozygous for both the disease and marker genotypes. However, it is not possible to establish phase unambiguously. It is not possible to know whether his D_1 allele is on the same chromosome as his M_1 or M_2 allele. So when calculating the likelihood for this family, it is necessary to include the uncertainty about phase by calculating the likelihood for the pedigree for each possible phase and weighting the resulting likelihoods by the probability of each phase. In this pedigree, there are two possible phases for the affected parent. Either the D_1 allele is on the same chromosome as the M_1 allele, which implies that the D_2 allele is on the same chromosome as the M_2 allele (call this phase I), or the D_1 allele is on the same chromosome as the M_2 allele, which implies that D_2 and M_1 are together (call this phase II).

The likelihood of the family in Figure 5-1 is calculated as follows: First, if the affected parent (I-1) is in phase I, then all of the offspring have received the parental combination of alleles from him and are nonrecombinants. If θ is the probability of recombination, then $1-\theta$ is the probability of nonrecombination. Or, in other words, $1-\theta$ is the probability that the gametes will be in the parental phase. Thus the likelihood of observing the sibship, assuming phase I for the affected parent, is $(1-\theta)^5$. If the affected parent is in phase II, then all of the offspring are recombinants and the likelihood of observing the family is θ^5. Combining these likelihoods and including the fact that phases I and II have equal a priori probability, the likelihood of this sibship is $L(\theta) = 0.5[(1 - \theta)^5 + \theta^5]$. Using this formulation, the likelihood for this family can be calculated for any value of the recombination fraction (θ).

As indicated above, linkage analysis consists of testing the null hypothesis of no linkage (θ = 0.5) by comparing its likelihood with the likelihood of alternative hypotheses of linkage (θ < 0.5) using the $\log_{10}$ of the odds ratio $L(\theta)/L(\theta = 0.5)$ (i.e., by calculating the lod score). For this pedigree, the lod score is given by $\log_{10}(16) + \log_{10}[(1 - \theta)^5 + \theta^5]$. [*Note:* $\log_{10}(16) = \log_{10}[(1 - \theta)^5 + \theta^5]$ for $\theta = 0.5$.] For $\theta = 0.0$, the lod score equals $\log_{10}(16) + 0 = 1.2$; for $\theta = 0.01$, the lod score equals $\log_{10}(16) = \log_{10}[(0.99)^5 + (0.01)^5] = 1.2 - 0.02 = 1.18$; for $\theta = 0.05$, lod $= 1.09$; and for $\theta = 0.10$, lod $= 0.97$.

While the calculation of the lod score for this small pedigree is straightforward, the task of calculating the lod score for families in which the genotypes are more variable or the size is larger is quite laborious. For example, suppose individual I-2 is heterozygous (M_1M_2) at the marker locus. Then for each individual in generation II, the calculation of the likelihood must take into account the probability that a haplotype (the combination of D and M alleles from one parent) present in the offspring came from either the mother or the father. For example, consider individual II-1. Assume the father (I-1) is in phase I. If the haplotype D_1M_1 came from the mother, then the haplotype D_2M_2 came from the father and represents a parental combination (i.e., is a nonrecombinant). However, if the mother transmitted the haplotype D_1M_2 to II-1, then the haplotype D_2M_1 transmitted from the father is a recombinant. If the father is in phase II, then the possibilities described are reversed. The change of genotype of individual I-2 thus reduces the amount of information in this pedigree and results in a decrease in the maximum lod score obtained. If the marker genotype for I-2 is M_1M_2, then the lod scores are 0.60, 0.59, 0.54, 0.47 for = 0.0, 0.01, 0.05, and 0.10 respectively. Thus the change in one genotype can have dramatic effect on the evidence for linkage.

With the study of more and larger families, the effect of just one change in genotype is minimized. However, increasing the number and size of families makes calculation of the lod scores much more tedious and difficult. Fortunately, computer programs have been developed that make the task more manageable. Thus linkage studies are feasible and can provide strong evidence that genetic factors are important for the expression of some trait. In fact, the replicated demonstration of genetic linkage constitutes proof that a gene that confers susceptibility

LIMITATIONS OF THE LINKAGE APPROACH FOR PSYCHIATRIC DISORDERS

The use of linkage methodology for complex disorders can have several limitations. All of the foregoing examples assumed complete penetrance for the susceptibility locus and complete typing and phenotype information for all individuals in the pedigree. For psychiatric disorders, the underlying genetic mechanisms are not known. Furthermore, in those cases where the patterns of transmission within families are consistent with a single gene, the estimate of penetrance has always been less than 1.0. The ability to estimate correctly and thus detect linkage decreases dramatically when there is reduced penetrance. If penetrance is reduced from 1.0 to 0.8, 20% of the individuals with the susceptibility genotype will not manifest the disease. These individuals will have the genetic marker associated with the illness. Since the individuals are unaffected, however, it is not possible to determine if they have the susceptibility genotype or whether there has been a crossover between the susceptibility locus and the marker locus. It follows, then, that when there is reduced penetrance, it becomes more difficult to estimate accurately the strength of linkage. Likewise, the misspecification of other parameters of the genetic model for the disease results in inaccurate estimates of the strength of the linkage relationship (Clerget-Darpoux, Bonaiti-Pellic, & Hochez, 1986). Changes in gene frequency, penetrance estimates, and diagnostic criteria can affect the results of linkage analyses significantly.

To illustrate the effect of reduced penetrance and variable age at onset, analyses were done with the data from the pedigree in Figure 5–1 using the modified version of LIPED (Hodge et al., 1979). The results are shown in Table 5–1. As can be seen, allowing for reduced penetrance in the genetic model has the effect of weakening the evidence for linkage.

Misclassification of the phenotype or a change in diagnosis can also have dramatic effects on the results of linkage analyses. Results in

TABLE 5–1
Reduction in Lod Scores Resulting from Incorporation of Reduced Penetrance

	Recombination (θ)					
Penetrance	0.00	0.01	0.05	0.10	0.15	0.20
1.00	1.20	1.18	1.09	0.98	0.85	0.72
0.90	0.93	0.91	0.83	0.74	0.63	0.52
0.80	0.84	0.82	0.75	0.66	0.56	0.46
0.50	0.59	0.58	0.52	0.45	0.38	0.30

Table 5–2 illustrate the effect of a change in the diagnosis of individual II-5 (Figure 5–1). If II-5 is affected and his or her genotype is M_1M_1, then the evidence for linkage is significantly reduced. This results from the fact that the M_2 allele is the one associated with the illness in other affected members in this pedigree. Since II-5 does not carry this allele, if affected, II-5 represents a recombinant. Thus diagnostic validity is crucial. If a person is misdiagnosed as affected, the result can be lethal to any linkage study. In the example, if II-5 were incorrectly diagnosed as affected, all of the evidence for linkage would disappear.

Misspecification of marker genotype can also have a dramatic effect on linkage analyses. The results shown in Table 5–3 demonstrate the effect of a change in one genotype from M_1M_1 to M_1M_2 for one of the offspring in the pedigree in Figure 5–1 (II-5). Note that if the

TABLE 5–2
Reduction in Lod Scores Resulting from a Change in Phenotype of One Individual in the Pedigree

	Recombination (θ)					
Penetrance	0.00	0.01	0.05	0.10	0.15	0.20
1.00	$-\infty$	−1.80	−0.19	0.02	0.10	0.12
0.90	−1.58	−0.82	−0.25	−0.04	0.04	0.07
0.80	−1.39	−0.84	−0.31	−0.10	−0.02	0.02
0.50	−1.01	−0.79	−0.42	−0.23	−0.13	−0.08

TABLE 5-3
Reduction of Lod Scores Resulting from the Change of One Marker Genotype in the Pedigree

Penetrance	Recombination (θ)					
	0.00	0.01	0.05	0.10	0.15	0.20
1.00	$-\infty$	-1.80	-0.19	0.02	0.10	0.12
0.90	0.66	0.66	0.60	0.53	0.45	0.37
0.80	0.62	0.60	0.55	0.48	0.41	0.33
0.50	0.47	0.46	0.41	0.35	0.29	0.23

calculations are done assuming complete penetrance, this change in genotype results in the lod score's plunging to $-\infty$ at $\Theta = 0.0$, since the disease genotype of that individual is assumed to be D_1D_1 under the assumption of complete penetrance. However, when the model incorporates reduced penetrance (as was done in the analyses for Table 5–3), the disease genotype of II-5 could be heterozygous. This possibility results in there being only a moderate decrease in the lod score for this particular pedigree (compare results in Tables 5–1 and 5–3). Nevertheless, these analyses demonstrate the need for care in the typing of markers for use in genetic linkage studies. Misclassification of marker genotypes will affect the lod score analyses. In some cases, the effect can be quite dramatic.

As illustrated by the results in Table 5–2, consideration of diagnostic classifications is particularly important when studying psychiatric disorders. In most cases, there is a considerable range and overlap of symptomatology between diagnostic categories, and accurate diagnosis can be difficult. Furthermore, no pathognomonic biological, neuropsychological, or clinical tests exist for diagnosing a psychiatric disorder independently of its full phenotypic expression. Unlike many inherited neurological or metabolic disorders, the definition of the affected psychiatric phenotype relies solely on clinical observations.

This issue (the overlap of symptomatology between diagnostic categories) is particularly salient for the affective disorders, because there has been some disagreement about whether bipolar and unipolar affective disorders are etiologically distinct illnesses. In addition, it is evident from family studies of bipolar affective disorders that there is an even wider spectrum of affective symptomatology among the relatives of bipolar probands (Andreasen et al., 1987; Rice et al., 1987). Chronic hypomania, minor depression, and other affective illnesses occur with greater frequency among relatives of bipolar probands, indicating that these conditions may represent variant expressions of the illness within families.

It has been proposed that genetic linkage studies will be helpful in defining the range of symptoms associated with a specific psychiatric illness. That is, if the marker genotype of an individual is known and that marker is tightly linked to the disease-susceptibility allele, then there is a high probability that the phenotype of that individual represents a possible phenotype of the disease-susceptibility genotype. If linkage studies are used in this way, there must be a second phase of analyses in which the results of the first phase are replicated. Without replication in an independent sample, it is not possible to know whether the chosen diagnostic grouping in the first set of analyses reflects the range of symptomatology that is inherited in a larger set of families or simply is a chance finding resulting from maximizing the lod score. Until such time that a linkage relationship has been established unequivocally, it will be necessary to delineate how changes in diagnostic hierarchies affect the results of linkage analyses.

A related issue is the importance of new onsets of illness in previously unaffected family members. The effects of new onsets and of the use of alternative diagnostic hierarchies are indistinguishable because broader diagnostic groupings and new onsets both result in the inclusion as affected of persons who were previously considered to be unaffected.

Recent findings from the Amish Study (Egeland et al., 1990; Kelsoe et al., 1989; Pauls et al., 1991) demonstrate that the evidence for linkage to chromosome 11p15 markers is not as compelling as originally reported. The results are strongly influenced by two recent onsets of illness in the pedigree and by the diagnostic classification used in the analyses. Egeland and colleagues (1990) demonstrated that the inclusion of a new-onset affected individual could lead to a decrease in the lod score, even when that individual had a haplotype consistent with linkage to a chromosomal region. At the present time, it is not possible to determine to what extent the new findings are due to either (1) the fact that there may be no linkage of bipolar affective disorder to markers on chromosome 11 or (2) expected fluctuations in lod scores resulting from the changes in diagnostic status of individuals as either affected or unaffected.

CONCLUSION

As has been demonstrated, the use of linkage analyses in the study of psychiatric illnesses has some potential limitations. These limitations need not be considered fatal flaws, but rather should be viewed as examples of areas where particular care is needed in the genetic study of abnormal behavior. None of these problems is insurmountable. Reliability checks are needed for both clinical evaluations and molecular genetic typings to guard against false-positive diagnoses and typing errors. Furthermore, linkage studies need to be done in conjunction with family and epidemiologic studies. Population-based family studies can provide useful information about the spectrum of illness that is inherited and lead to better estimates of genetic model parameters for incorporation into the linkage analyses. Linkage studies done in the context of population-based research are more likely to be successful because the definitions of phenotype and the estimates of the genetic models obtained from epidemiologic samples are more likely to be closer to the truth.

REFERENCES

Andreasen, N. C., Rice, J., Endicott, J., Coryell, W., Grove, W. M., & Reich, T. (1987). Familial rates of affective disorder. A report from the National Institute of Mental Health Collaborative Study. *Archives of General Psychiatry, 44,* 461–469.

Baron, M., Risch, N., Hamburger, R., Mandel, B., Kushner, S., Newan, M., Drumer, D., & Belmaker, R. H. (1987). Genetic linkage between X-chromosome markers and bipolar affective illness. *Nature, 326,* 289–292.

Clerget-Darpoux, F., Bonaiti-Pellie, C., & Hochez, J. (1986). Effects of misspecifying genetic parameters in lod score analysis. *Biometrics, 42,* 393–400.

Detera-Wadleigh, S. D., Berrettini, W., Goldin, L. R., Boorman, D., Anderson, S., & Gershon, E. S. (1987). Close linkage of c-Harvey-ras-1 and the insulin gene to affective disorder is ruled out in three North American pedigrees. *Nature, 325,* 806–808.

Detera-Wadleigh, S. D., Goldin, L. R., Sherrington, R., Encio, I., de Miguel, C., Berrettini, W., Gurling, H., & Gershon, E. S. (1989). Exclusion of linkage to 5g11-13 in families with schizophrenia and other psychiatric disorders. *Nature, 340,* 391–393.

Egeland, J. A., Gerhard, D. S., Pauls, D. L., Sussex, J. N., Kidd, K. K., Allen, C. R., Hostetter, A. M., & Housman, D. E. (1987). Bipolar affective disorders linked to DNA markers on chromosome 11. *Nature, 325,* 783–787.

Egeland, J. A., Sussex, J. N., Endicott, J., Hostetter, A. M., Offord, D. R., Schwab, J. J., & Pauls, D. L. (1990). The impact of diagnoses on genetic linkage study for bipolar affective disorders among the Amish. *Psychiatric Genetics, 1,* 5–18.

Hodge, S. E., Morton, L. A., Tideman, S., Kidd, K. K., & Spence, M. A. (1979). Age of onset correction available for linkage analysis (LIPED). *American Journal of Human Genetics, 31,* 761.

Hodgkinson, S., Sherrington, R., Gurling, H., Marchbanks, R., Reeders, S., Mallet, J., McInnis, M., Petursson, H., & Brynjolfsson, J. (1987). Molecular genetic evidence for heterogeneity in manic depression. *Nature, 325,* 805–806.

Kelsoe, J. R., Ginns, E. I., Egeland, J. A., Gerhard, D. S., Goldstein, A. M., Bale, S. J., Pauls, D. L., Long, R. T., Kidd, K. K., Conte, G., Housman, D. E., & Paul, S. M. (1989). Reevaluation of the linkage relationship between chromosome 11p loci and the gene for bipolar affective disorder in the Old Order Amish. *Nature, 342,* 238–243.

Kennedy, J. L., Giuffra, L. A., Moises, H. W., Cavalli-Sforza, L. L., Pakstis, A. J., Kidd, J. R., Castiglione, C. M., Sjogren, B., Wetterburg, L., & Kidd, K. K. (1988). Evidence against linkage of schizophrenia to markers on chromosome 5 in a northern Swedish pedigree. *Nature, 336,* 167–170.

Mendlewicz, J., Simon, P., Sevy, S., Charon, F., Brocas, H., Legros, S., & Vassart, G. (1987). Polymorphic DNA marker on X-chromosome and manic depression. *Lancet, 1*(8544), 1230–1232.

Morton, N. E. (1956). Sequential tests for the detection of linkage. *American Journal of Human Genetics, 7,* 277–318.

Ott, J. (1991). *Analysis of human genetic linkage* (rev. ed.). Baltimore, MD: Johns Hopkins Press.

Ott, J. (1976). A computer program for linkage analyses of general human pedigrees. *American Journal of Human Genetics, 28*, 528.

Pauls, D. L., Gerhard, D. S., Lacy, L. G., Hostetter, A. M., Allen, C. R., Bland, S. D., LaBuda, M. C., & Egeland, J. A. (1991). Linkage of bipolar affective disorders to markers on chromosome 11p is excluded in a second lateral extension of Amish pedigree 110. *Genomics, 11,* 730–736.

Penrose, L. S. (1953). The general purpose sib-pair linkage test. *Annals of Eugenics, 18,* 120–124.

Rice, J., Reich, T., Andreasen, N. C., Van Eerdewegh, M., Fishman, R., Hirschfeld, R. M., & Klerman, G. L. (1987). The familial transmission of bipolar illness. *Archives of General Psychiatry, 44,* 441–447.

Sherrington, R., Brynjolfsson, J., Petursson, H., Potter, M., Dudleston, K., Barraclough, B., Wasmuth, J., Dobbs, M., & Gurling, H. (1988). Localization of a susceptibility locus for schizophrenia on chromosome 5. *Nature, 336,* 164–167.

St. Clair, D., Blackwood, D., Muir, W., Baille, D., Hubbard, A., Wright, A., & Evans, H. J. (1989). No linkage of chromosome 5q11-q13 markers to schizophrenia in Scottish families. *Nature, 340,* 391–393.

Suarez, B. K., Rice, J., & Reich, T. (1978). The generalized sib pair IBD distribution: Its use in the detection of linkage. *Annals of Human Genetics, 42,* 87–94.

6

Molecular Genetic Studies in Affective Illness

JULIEN MENDLEWICZ

Recent progress in molecular behavioral genetics has attracted much attention and provided a new insight into the nature–nurture controversy with regard to psychiatric disorders. Affective illness, including the various subtypes of depressive and manic syndromes, has been the subject of a considerable amount of research on the relative importance of hereditary and environmental factors (Mendlewicz & Rainer, 1977; Mendlewicz, 1988).

The identification and precise localization of a major vulnerability gene in the transmission of affective illness could lead to better phenotype characterization and insight into the genetic etiology of these mental disorders. One of the most promising methods to explore major single genetic transmission is based on the analysis of linkage, a method in which the degree of cosegregation between genetic markers is evaluated, including DNA polymorphisms and illness traits in informative pedigrees.

LINKAGE STUDIES WITH CLASSICAL MARKERS

A number of studies have reported that the O blood group is most frequently found in manic-depressive patients (Barker, Theillie, & Spielberger, 1961; Mendlewicz, 1988). The association between a blood group factor and a major psychosis, although poorly understood, may indicate that the ABO genotype plays a role in the predisposition to manic-depressive illness. Association between traits is not to be confused with linkage; that is, the proximity of two traits on the same chromosome, resulting in their dependent assortment during the process of meiosis. In this method, one tries to test a potential linkage relationship between a known genetic marker and a character that is known to be genetically determined, but has not yet been mapped on the chromosome. It has been successfully in the genetic study of several hereditary conditions, and recently to test the hypothesis of genetic linkage in manic-depressive illness. Linkage to human leukocyte antigens (HLAs) on chromosome 6 has been suggested for affective illness (Wirtkamp, Stancer, Persad, Flood, & Guttorsmen, 1981; Stancer et al., 1988) but not confirmed in other studies (Targum, Gershon, Van Eerdewegh, & Rogenline, 1979; Goldin, Clerget-Darpoux, & Gershon, 1982; Clerget-Darpoux, Goldin, & Gershon, 1982; Suarez, Rice, Crouse, & Reich, 1983). Reich, Clayton, and Winokur (1969) studied two large families assorting for color blindness (an X-linked recessive marker) and bipolar illness, while Mendlewicz, Fleiss, and Fieve (1972) reported on seven such families. In both studies, the marker and the illness failed to show independent assortment. Winokur and Tanna (1969) described three more families, assorting in a dependent fashion for manic-depressive illness and the Xg blood group (a dominant X-linked marker).

Mendlewicz and Fleiss (1974) were able to demonstrate close linkage between bipolar illness and both deutan and protan* color blindness in 17 informative pedigrees and the absence of such linkage in 11 unipolar pedigrees. Recent linkage data confirm a linkage relationship between color blindness and bipolar manic-depressive illness (Baron, 1977; Mendlewicz, Linkowski, Guroff, & van Praag, 1979; Del Zompo, Bocchetta, Goldin, & Corsini, 1984; Baron et al., 1987) and are at variance with the report of Gershon, Targum, Matthyse, and Bunney (1979), who did not find such a linkage. A more comprehensive study—part of the Biological Psychiatry Collaborative Program of the World Health Organization—was conducted in four collaborative centers (Bethesda, Basel, Brussels, and Copenhagen) on 16 informative families, and the overall results were consistent with the presence of linkage between bipolar illness and color blindness. Some

---

* Deutan color blindness is a deficiency of green perception; protan is a deficiency of red perception. The chromosomal loci of these two conditions are closely linked, but are not identical.

families showed an X-linked pattern of inheritance, while others did not; this last observation suggested the hypothesis of genetic heterogeneity in manic-depressive illness (Gershon et al., 1980; Mendlewicz, 1974).

A comprehensive analysis of linkage data from the available literature shows that X linkage between color blindness and bipolar illness is indeed demonstrated in a large sample of families despite the presence of genetic heterogeneity (Risch & Baron, 1982; Risch, 1989; Van Eerdewegh, 1989).

Figure 6–1 illustrates the distribution of deuteranopia and bipolar–unipolar disorders in successive generations of a family informative for the analysis of linkage between colors blindness and affective illness.

Mendlewicz, Linkowski, and Wilmotte (1980) reported a positive linkage between bipolar illness and glucose-6-phosphate dehydrogenase deficiency (G6PD), which is a genetic marker on the X chromosome. Recently, Del Zompo and colleagues (1984) studied two pedigrees for bipolar illness, color blindness, and G6PD deficiency, which is closely linked with color blindness on the X chromosome (Siniscalco, Filippi, & Latte, 1964). Their results are also consistent with X linkage in bipolar illness. Like Kruger, Turner, and Kidd (1982), Risch and Baron (1982) also suggested genetic heterogeneity to explain discrepancies in X-linkage studies.

Table 6–1 summarizes the sex distribution in first-degree relatives of bipolar probands in some recent studies, most of which show a clear

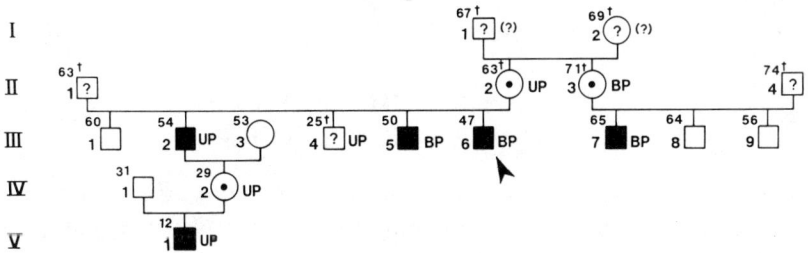

Figure 6–1. Pedigree indicative of X linkage of manic-depressive illness. UP = unipolar; BP = bipolar; ■ = male homozygous for deuteranpia; ⊙ = female heterozygous for deuteranopia; ? = male unknown status; (?) = female unknown status; ➤ = propositus.

TABLE 6-1
Percentage of Affectively Ill in First-Degree Relatives of Bipolar Patients

Study	Year	Total	Male(%)	Female(%)
Winokur & Crowe	1983	40	15(38)	25(63)
Mendlewicz & Rainer	1974	229	93(40)	136(60)
Winokur & Tanna	1969	76	20(26)	56(74)
Kadrmas et al.	1979	102	54(53)	48(47)
Stendstedt	1952	41	19(47)	22(53)
Angst et al.	1980	38	15(39)	23(61)
Mendlewicz & Rainer	1977	29	9(31)	20(69)
Gershon et al.	1978	79	38(48)	41(52)
Taylor & Abrams	1981	36	11(31)	25(69)
James & Chapman	1975	52	13(25)	39(75)
Goetzl et al.	1974	35	13(37)	22(63)
Gershon et al.	1975	36	20(55)	16(45)
Iowa Collaborative Study	1983	54	22(41)	32(59)
TOTAL		847	342(39)	505(61)

(From Winokur & Crowe (1983) see this reference for study citations.)

excess of females among the relatives of bipolar probands. However, other investigators have failed to find a preponderance of affected females, as compared with males, in first-degree relatives. Moreover, some family studies have shown a male-to-male transmission of the disease (Perris, 1968; Brown, Elston, Pollitzer, Prange, & Wilson, 1973; Goetzl, Green, Whybrow, & Jackson, 1974). Mendlewicz and Rainer (1974) observed the same phenomenon in about 10% of their overall sample, though it is nevertheless a rare event in the kindred of bipolar probands (Mendlewicz, 1985). Thus it seems quite clear that more that one genetic entity is involved in bipolar illness.

LINKAGE STUDIES WITH DNA MOLECULAR MARKERS

The DNA recombinant method and, more recently, the polymerase chain reaction (PCR) for gene amplification permit the exploration of DNA polymorphisms in various regions of the human genome (Bolstein, White, Skolnick, & Davis, 1980). Currently, linkage with DNA markers in manic-depressive disorder has been reported in two distinct chromosomal regions—the distal part of the short arm of chromosome 11 (11p15) and the subterminal region of the long arm of the X chromosome (Xq26-28).

Chromosome 11

Egeland et al. (1987), in studying a large pedigree of the Amish community, reported a positive linkage between manic-depressive disorder and the c-Harvey-ras-A (HRAS) oncogene, as well as the insulin (INS) marker on the short arm of chromosome 11. This linkage, however, could not be confirmed in American bipolar pedigrees of non-Amish origin (Detera-Wadleigh et al., 1987) and in other pedigrees of bipolar disorders (Hodgkinson et al., 1987; Gill, McKeon, & Humphries, 1988; Mitchell et al., 1991; Mendlewicz et al., 1991) as well as in pedigrees of unipolar disorder (Neiswanger et al., 1990; Wesner et al., 1990). Furthermore, a reanalysis of the original Amish pedigree with two unaffected subjects becoming ill in the core pedigree and including a lateral extension, could almost exclude the probability of linkage of affective illness to the 11p15 region of chromosome 11 (Kelsoe et al., 1989).

These apparently conflicting results perhaps could be explained on the following grounds: The vulnerability to affective illness could be linked to more than one gene (genetic heterogeneity), and this may also be the case in the extended family of the Amish isolate. Phenocopies may also be present in large pedigrees, especially for such common disorders as affective illness. Finally, the probability of localizing a major gene for affective disorder on this region of chromosome 11 is unlikely, despite the fact that the gene coding for tyrosine hydroxylase (TH) has been found to be closely linked to the INS and HRAS loci on chromosome 11. Studies of associations between the TH gene and affective illness have revealed positive results in one investigation (Leboyer et al., 1990), but this has not been confirmed in several other association studies (Todd & O'Malley, 1989; Körner, Fritze, & Propping, 1990). Another candidate gene located on the long arm of chromosome 11, the dopamine-2 receptor gene (D2) is also being explored because of the recent report of an association between a chromosomal translocation (region q21-22 of chromosome 11 and region q43 of chromosome 1) and psychiatric (including affective) disturbances in a large Scottish family (St. Clair et al., 1990).

Chromosome X

Previous linkage studies with classical X-chromosome markers have been confirmed by the finding of positive linkage between bipolar illness and the factor IX (hemophylia B) in region Xq27 in 10 Belgian pedigrees (Mendlewicz et al., 1987).

Negative linkage findings with DNA markers located in the color blindness and G6PD region (Xq28) have been reported by one group (Berrettini et al., 1990), but these results were obtained in a limited sample of small families with polymorphic psychiatric disturbances and few bipolar cases. They included the presence of affective illness on both the paternal and maternal sides, and apparent transmission of illness from father to son in several families, despite positive linkage scores for the ST-14 probe (Xq28 region) in two families, which renders these negative results less convincing.

An association between the fragile X syndrome and affective illness has also been observed (Pascalis, Teyssier, & Carre-Pigeon, 1985; Reiss et al., 1986) and recently was confirmed in one family (Mendlewicz & Hirsch, 1991). Another gene of interest in the Xq28 region is the gene of the α_3 subunit of the pi106-aminobutyric acid (GABA) receptor (GABRA^3) (Buckle et al., 1989), which makes it a candidate gene for the genetic study of manic-depressive disorder.

Thus the overall linkage data confirm the presence of a major locus of transmission of bipolar illness in the Xq27-28 region on the long arm of the X chromosome.

Table 6-2 summarizes the linkage studies of the X-linked form of bipolar illness.

Positive X-linkage results have been confirmed in 14 different samples on a total of 59 pedigrees collected in seven centers located in

TABLE 6-2
X-Linkage Studies of Bipolar Illness

	Pedigrees	Studies	Centers	Countries
Positive	59	14	7	United States (3) Israel (2) Belgium (1) Italy (1)
Negative	14	2		United States

various countries, including the United States ($n = 3$), Israel ($n = 2$), Belgium ($n = 1$), and Italy ($n = 1$).

The prevalence rate of the X-linked form of bipolar illness in the general population and its clinical phenotypical characteristics remain to be defined. Some data suggest that X-linked bipolar affective illness may be associated with an early onset (before age 30) (Mendlewicz & Simon, 1987); (Baron et al., 1990), a greater psychiatric morbidity as suggested by an increased relapse rate, and a greater loading of bipolar disorders in relatives (Baron et al., 1990).

As for unipolar illness, chromosomal linkage studies have so far rejected the presence of a locus on chromosome X and chromosome 11 in this affective disorder (Mendlewicz & Fleiss, 1974; Neiswanger et al., 1990; Wesner et al., 1990).

CONCLUSIONS

The X-linked form of bipolar illness has now been substantiated by several family studies and numerous linkage studies using classical and DNA markers in the Xq27-28 region of the X chromosome. Non-X-linked forms of the illness are most likely to be present (genetic heterogeneity), but the transmission of a major susceptibility gene on the short arm of chromosome 11 has not been confirmed. The linkage strategy so far has been inconclusive in the search for a single gene transmission model (Mendlewicz & Fleiss, 1974; Hill, Wilson, Felston, & Winokur, 1988; Wesner et al., 1990; Neiswanger et al., 1990) in unipolar depression, but the heterogeneity and phenocopies are probably much more present in the unipolar forms of affective illness.

The identification and separation of genetic subgroups of the affective disorders with the use of genetic markers and candidate genes could allow a better clinical, biochemical, and therapeutic approach to these complex behavioral disorders. Caution should be taken to avoid making premature claims of linkage because of the possibility of spurious linkage when dealing with selective ascertainment of frequent disorders and common genetic markers, as seems to be the case in the area of psychiatric disorders. The study of the interaction between genetic and nongenetic vulnerability factors remains a major challenge for future research strategies in the affective illness.

REFERENCES

Barker, J. B., Theillie, A., & Spielberger, C. D. (1961). Frequency of blood types in a homogenous group of manic-depressive patients. *Journal of Mental Sciences, 107,* 936–942.

Baron, M. (1977). Linkage between an X-chromosome marker (deutan color blindness) and bipolar affective illness. *Archives of General Psychiatry, 34,* 721–725.

Baron, M., Hamburger, R., Sandkuyl, L. A., Risch, N., Mandel, B., Endicott, J., Belmaker, R. H., & Ott, J. (1990). The impact of phenotypic variation of genetic analysis: Application to X-linkage in manic-depressive illness. *Acta Psychiatrica Scandinavica, 82,* 196–203.

Baron, M., Risch, N., Hamburger, R., Mandel, B., Kushner, S., Newman, M., & Belmaker, R. H. (1987). Genetic linkage between X-chromosome markers and bipolar affective illness. *Nature, 326,* 289–292.

Berrettini, W. H., Goldin, L. R., Gelernter, J., Gesman, P. V., Gershon, E. S., & Detera-Wadleigh, S. D. (1990). X-chromosome markers and manic-depressive illness: Rejection of linkage to XQ28 in nine bipolar pedigrees. *Archives of General Psychiatry, 47,* 366–373.

Bolstein, D., White, R. L., Skolnick, M., & Davis, R. W. (1980). Construction of a genetic linkage map in man using restriction fragment length polyporphism. *American Journal of Human Genetics, 32,* 314–331.

Brown, R. J., Elston, R. C., Pollitzer, W. S., Prange, A., & Wilson, E. (1973). Sex-ratio in relatives of patients with affective disorder. *Biological Psychiatry, 6,* 307–309.

Buckle, V. J., Fujita, N., Ryder-Cook, A. S., Derrz, J., Barnard, P. J., Lebo, R. V., Schofield, P. R., Seeburg, P. H., Bateson, A. N., Darlison, M. G., & Barnard E. A. (1989). Chromosomal localization of GABA A receptor subunit genes, relationship to human genetic disease. *Neuron, 3,* 647–654.

Clerget-Darpoux, F., Goldin, L. R., & Gershon, E. S. (1982). A new method for analysis of HLA-associated diseases. *American Journal of Human Genetics, 35,* 127–130.

Del Zompo, M., Bocchetta, A., Goldin, L. R., & Corsini, G. U. (1984). Linkage between X-chromosome markers and manic-depressive illness in two Sardinian pedigrees. *Acta Psychiatrica Scandinavica, 70,* 282–287.

Detera-Wadleigh, S. D., Berrettini, W. H., Goldin, L. R., Boorman, D., Anderson, S., & Gershon, E. S. (1987). Close linkage of C-Harvey-ras-1 and the insulin gene to affective disorder is ruled out in three North American pedigrees. *Nature, 325,* 806–807.

Egeland, J. A., Gerhard, D. S., Paul, D. C., Sussex, J. N., Kidd, K. K., Allen, C. R., Hostetter, A. M., & Housman, D. E. (1987). Bipolar affective disorder linked to DNA markers on chromosome 11. *Nature, 325,* 783–787.

Gershon, E. S., Mendlewicz, J., Gastpar, M., Bech, P., Goldin, L. R., Kielholz, P., Rafaelsen, O. J., Vartanian, F., & Bunney, W. E., Jr. (1980). WHO collaborative study of genetic linkage of bipolar manic-depressive illness and red/green color blindness. *Acta Psychiatrica Scandinavica, 61,* 319–338.

Gershon, E. S., Targum, S. D., Matthyse, S., & Bunney, W. E., Jr. (1979). Color blindness not closely linked to bipolar illness. *Archives of General Psychiatry, 36,* 1423–1431.

Gill, M., McKeon, P., & Humphries, P. (1988). Linkage analysis of manic-depression in an Irish family using H-ras 1 and INS DNA markers. *Journal of Medical Genetics, 25,* 634–637.

Goetzl, V., Green R., Whybrow, P., & Jackson, R. (1974). X-linkage revisited. A further family study of manic-depressive illness. *Archives of General Psychiatry, 31,* 665–672.

Goldin, L. R., Clerget-Darpoux, F., & Gershon, E. S. (1982). Relationship of HLA to major affective disorders not supported. *Psychiatry Research, 7,* 28–45.

Hill, E., Wilson, A. F., Felston, R. C., & Winokur, G. (1988). Evidence for possible linkage between genetic markers and affective disorders. *Biological Psychiatry, 24,* 903–917.

Hodgkinson, S., Sherrington, R., Gurling, H., Marchbanks, M., Reeders, S., Mallet, J., McInnis, M., Petursson, H., & Brynjolfsson, J. (1987). Molecular genetic evidence of heterogeneity in manic-depression. *Nature, 325,* 805–806.

Kelsoe, J. R., Ginns, E. I., Egeland, J. A., Gerhard, D. S., Golstein, A. M., Bale, S. J., Pauls, D. L., Long, R. J., Kidd, K. K., Conte, G., Housman, D. E., & Paul, S. M. (1989). Re-evaluation of the linkage relationship between chromosome 11p loci and the gene for bipolar affective disorder in the Old Order Amish. *Nature, 342,* 238–243.

Körner, J., Fritze, J., & Propping, P. (1990). RFLP alleles at the tyrosine hydroxylase locus: No association found to affective disorders. *Psychiatry Research, 32,* 275–280.

Kruger, S. D., Turner, J. W., & Kidd, K. K. (1982). The effects of requisite assumptions on linkage analyses of manic-depressive illness with HLA. *Biological Psychiatry, 17,* 1081–1099.

Leboyer, M., Malafosse, A., Boularand, S., Campion, D., Gheeysen, F., Samolyk, D., Henriksson, B., Denise, E., Des Lauriers, A., Lepine, J.

P., Zarifian, E., Clerget-Darpoux, F., & Mallet, J. (1990). Tyrosine hydroxylase polymorphisms associated with manic-depressive illness. *Lancet, 335,* 1219.

Mendlewicz, J. (1974). Le concept d hétérogénéité dans la psychose maniaco-dépressive. *L' évolution Psychiatrique, 2,* 411–416.

Mendlewicz, J. (1985). X-linked inheritance in affective disorders. In P. Pichot, P. Berner, R. Wolf, & K. Thau (Eds.), *Psychiatry* (vol. 2, pp. 95–99). New York: Plenum.

Mendlewicz, J. (1988). Population and family studies in depression and mania. *British Journal of Psychiatry, 153* (suppl. 3), 16–25.

Mendlewicz, J., & Fleiss J. L. (1974). Linkage studies with X-chromosome markers in bipolar (manic-depressive) and unipolar depressive illness. *Biological Psychiatry, 9,* 261–294.

Mendlewicz, J., Fleiss, J., & Fieve, R. R. (1972). Evidence for X-linkage in the transmission of manic-depressive illness. *JAMA, 222* (13), 1624–1627.

Mendlewicz, J., & Hirsch, D. (1991). Fragile X syndrome and manic-depression. *Biological Psychiatry, 29,* 295–308.

Mendlewicz, J., Leboyer, M., Malafosse A., Sevy, S., Hirsch, D., Babron, M. C., van Broeckhoven, C., & Mallet J. (1991). No linkage between chromosome 11p15 markers and manic-depressive illness in a Belgian pedigree. *American Journal of Psychiatry, 148* (12), 1683–1687.

Mendlewicz, J., Linkowski, P., Guroff, J. J., & van Praag, H. M. (1979). Color-blindness linkage to bipolar manic-depressive illness. New evidence. *Archives of General Psychiatry, 36,* 1442–1447.

Mendlewicz, J., Linkowski, P., & Wilmotte, J. (1980). Linkage between glucose-6-phosphate dehydrogenase deficiency and manic-depressive psychosis. *British Journal of Psychiatry, 137,* 337–342.

Mendlewicz, J., & Rainer, J. (1974). Morbidity risk and genetic transmission in manic-depressive illness. *American Journal of Human Genetics, 26,* 692–701.

Mendlewicz, J., & Rainer, J. (1977). Adoption study supporting genetic transmission in manic-depression illness. *Nature, 268,* 327–329.

Mendlewicz, J., & Simon, P. (1987). Linkage analysis in manic-depressive illness. *Lancet, 2,* (855)4, 345.

Mendlewicz, J., Simon, P., Sevy, S., Charon, F., Brocas, H., Legros, S., & Vassart, G. P. (1987). Polymorphic DNA marker on X-chromosome and manic-depression. *Lancet, 2,* 1230–1232.

Mitchell, P., Wraters, B., Morrison, N., Shine, J., Donald, J., & Eisman, J. (1991). Close linkage of bipolar disorder to chromosome 11 markers is excluded in two large Australian pedigrees. *Journal of Affective Disorders, 21,* 23–32.

Neiswanger, K., Slaugenhaulst, S. A., Hughes, H. B., Frank, E., Frankel, D. R., McCarthy, M. I., Chakravarti, A., Zubenko, G. S., Kupfer, D. J., & Kaplan, B. B. (1990). Evidence against close linkage of unipolar affective illness to human chromosome 11p markers HRAS 1 and INS and chromosome Xq marker DX552. *Biological Psychiatry, 28,* 63–72.

Pascalis, G., Teyssier, J. R., & Carre-Pigeon, F. (1985). Présence d 'un Xq-Fra chez un maniaque, situation du géne de la P.M.D. sur le bras long du chromosome X. *Annals Medico-Psycholoqiques, 146,* 594–595.

Perris, C. (1968). Genetic transmission of depressive psychoses. *Acta Psychiatrica Scandinavica, 203* (suppl.), 45–52.

Reich, T., Clayton, P. J., & Winokur, G. (1969). Family history study in the genetics of mania. *American Journal of Psychiatry, 125,* 1358–1359.

Reiss, A. L., Feinstein, C., Toomey, K. E., Goldsmith, B., Rosenbaum, K., & Caruso, M. A. (1986). Psychiatric disability associated with the fragile X-chromosome. *American Journal of Medical Genetics, 23,* 394–401.

Risch, N. (1989). Description of X-linkage pedigrees. *Genetic Epidemiology, 6,* 187–189.

Risch, N., & Baron, M. (1982). X-linkage and genetic heterogeneity in bipolar related major affective illness: Re-analysis of linkage data. *Annals of Human Genetics, 46,* 153–166.

St. Clair, D., Blackwood, D., Muir, W., Carothers, A., Walkers, M., Spowart, G., Gosden, C., & Evans, H. J. (1990). Association within a family of a balanced autosomal translocation with mental illness. *Lancet, 336,* 13–16.

Siniscalco, M., Filippi, G., & Latte, B. (1964). Recombination between protan and deutan genes: Data on their relative positions in respect of the G6PD locus. *Nature, 204,* 1061–1064.

Stancer, H. C., Weitkamp, L. R., Persad, E., Flood, C., Jorna, T., Guttorsmen, S. A., & Yagnow, R. L. (1988). Confirmation of the relationship of HLA (chromosome 6) genes to depression and manic-depression. *Annals of Human Genetics, 52,* 279–298.

Suarez, B. K., Rice, J. P., Crouse, J., & Reich, T. (1983). HLA and disease: Haplotype sharing in multiflex families. *Clinical Genetics, 23,* 267–275.

Targum, S. D., Gershon, E. J., Van Eerdewegh, M., & Rogenline, N., (1979) Human leucocytes antigen (HLA) system not closely linked to or associated with bipolar manic-depressive illness. *Biological Psychiatry, 14,* 615–636.

Todd, R., & O'Malley, K. (1989). Population frequencies of tyrosine hydroxylase RFLP in bipolar affective disorders. *Biological Psychiatry, 25,* 626–630.

Van Eerdewegh, P. (1989). Linkage analysis with cohort effects: An application to X-linkage. *Genetic Epidemiology, 6,* 271–276.

Wesner, R. B., Tanna, V. L., Palmer, P. J., Goedken, R. J., Crowe, R. R., & Winokur, G. (1990). Linkage of c-Harvey-ras-1 and INS DNA markers to unipolar depression and alcoholism is ruled out in 18 families. *European Archives of Psychiatric Neurological Sciences, 239,* 356–360.

Winokur, G., & Crowe, R. R. (1983). Bipolar illness, the sex-polarity effects in affectively ill family members. *Archives of General Psychiatry, 40,* 57–58.

Winokur, G., & Tanna, V. L. (1969). Possible role of X-linked dominant factor in manic-depressive disease. *Diseases of the Nervous System, 30,* 89–93.

Wirtkamp, L. R., Stancer, H. C., Persad, E., Flood, C., & Guttorsmen, S. (1981). Depressive disorders and HLA. A gene on chromosome 6 that can affect behavior. *New England Journal of Medicine, 305,* 1301–1306.

PART II
Clinical Aspects of the Genetic Studies

7

The Family Psychoeducational Approach
Rationale for a Multigenerational Treatment Modality for the Major Affective Disorders

DEMITRI F. PAPOLOS

Seymour Kety's classical study (Kety et al., 1968), which followed parents and their adopted and biological offspring in Denmark, provided evidence that schizophrenia has a hereditary component. He also provided a methodology that has since been used to study other psychiatric disorders, including manic-depressive illness. Twenty years ago, the idea of a genetic influence on complex human behavior was anathema to many, and the findings from Kety's studies were met with great resistance, not only from a large segment of the public, but from many behavioral scientists and psychiatrists who maintained that such behavioral disorders must be due primarily to environmental factors. The acceptance of genetics as an important factor in mental illness has come slowly. In retrospect, it is not difficult to ask how anyone could have doubted the mounting evidence. Yet, while the

---

Supported by National Institute of Mental Health Physician Scientist Research Development Award 1K20MH00873-01A2 and by a NARSAD Young Investigator Award.

implications of the emerging genetic data largely substantiate the importance of a genetically transmitted vulnerability for mood disorders and schizophrenia, they also point to the importance of environmental factors.

Major affective disorders are familial illnesses. The biological relatives of both unipolar and bipolar patients are at far greater risk than the general population for developing affective illness. Familial is, of course, not synonymous with genetic, but several lines of evidence converge on attributing a major portion of this increased familial incidence to genetic factors (Bertelsen, Harvald, & Hauge, 1977; Mendlewicz & Rainer, 1977). The similar rates of mood disorders in every race, culture, and geographic location has bolstered the idea that these conditions have a genetic basis (Boyd & Weissman, 1981). Over the past half-century, numerous twin adoptions, and family studies all suggested that genetic factors were important in the etiology of mood disorders. Twin studies support the general case for a genetic factor but fail to tease apart the interactions between heredity and environment (Bertelson et al., 1977). Although adoption studies attempt more clearly to separate the influence of nature versus nurture and again attest to a genetic factor, they also indicate that the disorder is not wholly genetic (Mendlewicz & Rainer, 1977). Approximately a third of identical twins reared apart are not concordant for the disorder, suggesting that environmental factors also interact in some way with the genetic trait.

The most compelling evidence for genetic influence on a particular illness, short of finding the mutant allele, is to establish linkage to a known genetic marker—two traits segregating together in families because the genes that determine the two traits are located near one another on a chromosome. Unfortunately, as will be described in this book, obtaining evidence for linkage to known markers is handicapped by the complexities of psychiatric disorders. The simple Mendelian models—autosomal dominant, X-linked dominant, and recessive—must be modified to account for nongenetic factors. Confounding factors, such as age-related penetrance, variable presentations of illness within the same families, and lack of consensus diagnoses, have thus far precluded the development of a working genetic model (Faraone, Kreman, & Tsuang, 1990) (also see Chapters 2 and 5).

THE GENERATIONAL IMPACT OF MOOD DISORDERS

When a parent is affected with a mood disorder, there is strong evidence of a markedly increased risk of childhood disorders in their offspring (Beardslee, Bemporad, Keller, & Klerman, 1983; Beardslee, Keller, & Klerman, 1985). Children who have at least one parent with an affective disorder have a significantly increased rate of depression and other psychopathology when compared with children whose parents have no history of affective illness (Akiskal et al., 1985; Weissman et al., 1987; Weissman, Warner, Wickramaratne, & Prusoff, 1988). In a study of the offspring of parents with manic-depressive illness which used direct interviews with children, Decina and colleagues (1983) found an increased frequency of major and minor affective disorders in children of bipolar parents as compared with normal controls. Hammen, Burge, Burney, and Adrian (1990) reported on offspring from four groups of mothers, including unipolar, bipolar, medically ill, and normal mothers. This study found that the children in the two affective disorder parent groups had very high rates of diagnoses (82% unipolar, 72% bipolar). Offspring of the medical group had lower (43%) but nonetheless moderate rates compared with children in the normal group (22%). It is apparent from offspring research, both cross-sectional and longitudinal, that when a parent is ill, the children are likely to also manifest some psychiatric disorder. Thus mood disorders are not illnesses that affect just individuals; they are also familial illnesses that may have lifelong consequences across multiple generations.

Many family studies not only have found higher rates of bipolar disorder among relatives of bipolar probands, but also increased rates of major depression and other forms of affective illness (Perris, 1966; Tsuang & Faraone, 1990). Wender et al. (1986), investigating the contribution of genetic and environmental factors to the etiology of mood disorders, found an eight-fold increase in unipolar depression and a 15-fold increase in suicide among the biological relatives of index cases with unipolar depression. This study demonstrated a significant genetic contribution to unipolar depression and suicide. Studies have shown that more than 25% of patients with unipolar affective disorder have a parent or first-degree relative with an affective disorder. Taken together, these findings are compelling justification for clinical interventions that undertake to evaluate and treat the family.

While the evidence for a genetic contribution to the etiology of these disorders is beyond dispute, none of the studies indicates that genetic effects account for all the variation between ill and not ill individuals. Indeed, when viewed objectively, the genetic data also support substantial effects of environmental influences on the development of illness. Because of the increased risk in these families, the genetic vulnerability to develop affective illness is compounded by loss during childhood through parental illness, suicide, separation, divorce, or more subtle forms of emotional deprivation (Davenport, Adland, Gold, & Goodwin, 1979).

Studies that have examined the effects on children raised by affectively ill parents have found that deficits in maternal parenting increase the offspring's risk of developing impairments in mood regulation and social relations, as well as for other psychiatric conditions (Davenport, Zahn-Waxler, Adland, & Mayfield, 1983; Zahn-Waxler, Cummings, & McKnew, 1984; Hammen et al., 1987a,b). Kochanska and colleagues (1987) compared normal, unipolar, and bipolar depressed mothers to determine whether depressive cognitive schemas extend to the perception of one's own child. Compared with well mothers, women from the depressed groups were less satisfied with their children's social and emotional development, experienced more helplessness regarding their offspring, and were more likely to feel that outcomes of their child's development would be determined by uncontrollable factors. Hammen et al., (1987b), in one of the few high-risk studies to investigate the impact of the variable of chronic stress in association with maternal depression, found that chronic family stress and current maternal depressive symptoms were more predictive of children's behavioral dysfunction than was a history of maternal affective illness.

Recent findings from an examination of data derived from the Amish Study further support the role of nongenetic maternal influences on the development of mood disorders. Carter and colleagues (1992) found that the offspring of affectively ill mothers and affectively ill fathers were at similar high risk when the parental psychiatric disorder was severe, for example, bipolar I disorder. However, when the parental affective illness was less severe, the offspring of affected mothers were at greater risk for illness than the offspring of affected fathers. Since there is no difference in the rate of affective illness among all relatives of male and female probands in the Amish community, they conclude that the family environment influences the expression of the underlying genetic vulnerability.

In recent decades, there has been a progressive increase in lifetime rates of major depression in the general population (Klerman et al., 1985; Gershon et al., 1985, 1987b). The increase is especially marked in the late teen and early adult years. These newly reported findings from epidemiologic studies of cohorts born after 1940 have rather ominous public-health implications. It is anticipated that as the younger cohorts age in the coming decades, a lifetime hazard of a broad spectrum of affective disorders will be observed that is greatly in excess of that observed in the previous generations. These studies also identify a population at greatly increased risk: the families of patients with affective disorders (Klerman et al., 1985).

Gershon and colleagues (1987b) suggested that one explanation for their finding of increased risk to later generations could be an increase in affective disorders in U.S. metropolitan areas that is due to nongenetic factors. One possible explanation for an earlier age of onset of affective disorder would be exposure at an early age (during childhood) to a parent who is experiencing affective illness, and consequently altering the dynamics of the family rearing situation. Stancer and colleagues (1987) examined this possibility in a study that compared the morbidity risk for affective disorder in relatives of probands who had bipolar disorder or major depression. Their review of the relatives of younger-onset patients revealed that 28% of the 128 siblings and 28% of the 40 offspring had developed affective disorder. On the other hand, 26% of 90 siblings and only 19% of 59 offspring of probands had later onset developed affective disorder. Therefore, the effect of age of onset of the probands is demonstrated—the increase in risk to relatives of younger-onset patients is for offspring, not siblings. An earlier age of onset of affective illness (in general, before the age of 40) increases the risk for all types of mood disorders among relatives, regardless of sex of proband or relative (Rice et al., 1987; Tsuang & Faraone, 1990). Additionally, there appears to be a particularly strong hereditary component in adolescent-onset affective illness. For example, patients with adolescent-onset bipolar disorders are associated with a rate of mood disorders or any psychiatric illness in first-degree relatives of 33% and 58%, respectively (Strober & Carlson, 1982). In this study, adolescent-onset unipolar depression carried a lesser but likewise significant risk to first-degree relatives, 25% and 47% respectively. As many of the proband's siblings were quite young, and had not passed through the period of risk for illness, these rates of risk are likely to increase significantly over time.

GENETIC FINDINGS—IMPLICATIONS FOR CLINICAL ASSESSMENT AND TREATMENT

The findings that inheritance patterns suggestive of greater genetic deviance (i.e., loaded, multigenerational, and bipolar 1–positive pedigrees) are predictive of bipolar outcome lend support to the idea that much can be foretold about the diagnosis and subsequent course of illness in juveniles from the degree of affective morbidity in their family pedigree. These findings have implications for researchers interested in the ascertainment of pedigrees for linkage studies, as well as for clinical diagnosis and for the development of preventive treatment approaches.

Increasingly, retrospective diagnostic surveys are finding that patients with an earlier onset of affective illness in adolescence, especially if the initial hospitalization was for mania, are far more likely to receive a diagnosis of schizophrenia (Joyce, 1984). Unfortunately, the misdiagnosis of psychotic forms of mood disorders is not at all uncommon within the general patient population (Pope & Lipinski, 1983). This is of great clinical significance, since prospective, longitudinal, and retrospective analyses of the course of illness indicate that early and effective intervention with appropriate somatic treatments may have a pronounced effect on long-term outcome and cycle frequency (Prien et al., 1984; Prien & Kupfer, 1986; Baastrup & Schou, 1967; Angst, Weis, Grof, Baastrup, & Schou, 1970; Post & Weiss, 1989). In addition, patients whose bipolar illness began during adolescence are reported to present with a predominance of psychotic symptomatology (Strober & Carlson, 1982). Since there is no established pattern of illness, the diagnosis of psychotic disorders in this age group is fraught with uncertainty. Clinicians who rely only on the acute presentation of symptoms are much more likely to misdiagnose these patients as schizophrenic. While it is not universally the case, these conditions tend to breed true. In support of this notion, Egeland (personal communication) has observed that in the 37 multigenerational bipolar pedigrees ascertained by the Amish Study, no first-degree relative in this sample of 404 individuals was diagnosed by the psychiatric board (blind to family history) as having schizophrenia. Therefore, a positive family history of affective disorders in first-degree relatives may be of great clinical significance in diagnostic deliberations in this age group, and provides further justification for the inclusion of the family in the diagnostic process. This is of practical importance for several reasons: when misdiagnosed, the patient is likely to be denied a trial on medication more suitable for affective disorders, and with inappropriate treatment, the likelihood of chronicity or relapsing affective episodes is much greater. The practical importance of determining predictors of bipolar illness during the period of adolescence is underscored by follow-up data that suggest that the onset of bipolar disorder in early adolescence may portend an especially malignant outcome with a high incidence of suicide and frequent, recurring mood swings, presumably because uncontrolled fluctuations in the affective state have concomitant long-term effects on personality development (Strober et al., 1988).

Given the fact that the vulnerability to develop an affective disorder is inherited and that these disorders frequently are not accurately identified, and often are undertreated even when correctly diagnosed, coupled with the public-health implications of the recent epidemiologic studies (Gershon et al., 1987b; Klerman et al., 1985), it is clear that the establishment of educational programs directed toward high-risk families will be of critical importance over the next several decades.

CURRENT TREATMENT STRATEGIES— DO THEY REFLECT THE CURRENT STATE OF KNOWLEDGE?

Major affective disorders continue to be the leading causes of psychiatric disability, loss of productivity, consumption of health resources, and human suffering (Baldessarini, 1983; Prien & Kupfer, 1986). While the great majority of major depressions are recurrent, alternate or mix with excited psychotic states, or may become chronic (Baldessarini & Tohen, 1988), historically, the recurrent nature of these illnesses has been underestimated by American psychiatric researchers and clinical practitioners (Goodwin, 1989). Thus the need to develop safe, effective, and efficient long-term treatments for these disorders is of extreme importance.

Within the past decade, the thrust of the community mental health movement at the national and local level has generated a treatment model for the major psychiatric disorders composed of two phases—a brief inpatient plan measured in weeks, followed by an extended period of aftercare in the community. The knowledge base that would help to develop a firm relationship between treatment methods and the prevention of relapse following an acute episode of depression or mania has only been thinly developed, particularly in the case of integrated treatment strategies that are shaped and guided by psychological, biological, and environmental factors. These factors have been poorly understood and rarely studied interactively.

While most studies of drug-treatment response have focused on the effect on acute episodes of illness, during the past five years, clinical and research interest in the affective disorders has expanded beyond the diagnosis and treatment of acute episodes to include consideration of long-term maintenance treatment aimed at prevention or reduction of the frequency and intensity of further attacks. This interest in preventive treatment has been largely stimulated by results from long-term drug trials with antidepressants and lithium primarily designed to examine the comparative effects of different pharmacological treatments (Schou, 1979; Kukopulos & Reginaldi, 1980; Keller, Lavori, Rice, Coryell, & Hirschfeld, 1986), as well as the mounting realization that these conditions are, in a large proportion of cases, recurrent (Zis & Goodwin, 1979; Kukopulos, Reginaldi, Laddomada et al., 1980; Goodwin, 1989).

Unfortunately, very few well-controlled studies have systematically evaluated the impact of these illnesses on long-term psychological and interpersonal function or considered their impact on the family. As a result, a number of core questions have remained unanswered as to the implementation of effective models of treatment following hospital discharge. What are the factors that contribute to relapse and rehospitalization? What role does the patient's and family's understanding of the nature and course of illness play in the patient's adherence to a maintenance treatment program? What is the effect of episodes of illness on other family members? These questions are particularly pressing in the case of the major affective disorders given the natural course of these illnesses, with such heavy family loading, propensity for relapse and recurrence, and clear attendant consequences for the subsequent generation at risk.

Mood disorders affect one in five families. Of patients requiring acute psychiatric hospitalization, surveys have shown that clearly one-third to one-half have some form of affective disorder and are often underdiagnosed (Keisling, 1981). Treatment in most inpatient settings is brief and usually focuses on the management of acute symptoms. Once stabilized, patients are often discharged with little or no information about the nature of their condition and the implications for treatment. In a recent survey of 80 patients diagnosed with bipolar affective disorder (manic-depressive disease) admitted consecutively to the inpatient service of a municipal hospital in New York City (most with at least two previous psychiatric hospitalizations for mania or depression), over 90% of patients and 98% of the family members interviewed were unaware of their diagnosis (Papolos, unreported observations). An equal number did not know that they would be expected to continue on lithium for the rest of their lives.

Mental health professionals have often avoided detailed discussions of diagnosis, symptoms, and prognosis. Commonly held reasons for doing so include lack of diagnostic clarity, the ill effects of stigmatization, discomfort with imparting such information, and the potentially harmful effects of a distressed reaction on the part of the individual with the illness (Tsuang & Vandermey, 1980). The evidence from studies in general medical settings and lithium clinics suggests that by failing to educate the patient and family, physicians may inadvertently contribute to medication noncompliance that leads to relapse and rehospitalization (Jamison & Akiskal, 1983). It is important to note that psychiatrists can serve patients and their families beyond offering risk estimates: they can dispel myths surrounding the illness and increase the stability of the family environment by decreasing the family members' anxiety about the patient and increasing their self-confidence and knowledge about the disorder. Knowledge is empowering and can improve the family's capacity to react constructively to those who are affected. Psychoeducational approaches for various forms of psychiatric illness have resulted in significantly reduced relapse rates following acute episodes of illness and a markedly increased compliance with treatment (Anderson, Hogarty, & Reiss, 1986).

While the evidence to support the belief that the vulnerability to develop a major affective disorder is genetically transmitted and neurochemically expressed has been strengthened over the past decade, it has unfortunately been accompanied by a philosophy that drugs and other somatic therapies offer the best, and sometimes the only, choice for treatment. This view of what comprises adequate treatment is short-sighted. There is currently no evidence to support strict adherence to a purely psychotherapeutic or purely pharmacological treatment strategy. Indeed, there is some evidence to support the idea that pharmacological treatment alone is not sufficient to prevent relapse in a large percentage of cases (e.g., Rounsaville, Prusoff, & Weissman, 1980; Frank & Kupfer, 1986; Frank et al., 1990). Simply relegating these disorders to the realm of physiological disturbances that require medical treatment alone is a serious clinical oversight and a gross scientific presumption, similar to the earlier psychological oversimplifications and prejudices that compounded the difficulties that have inhibited the development of multidimensional treatment approaches.

MOOD DISORDERS—THE IMPACT ON THE FAMILY

The onset of a chronic, relapsing illness in a family is a major source of unremitting stress for every member of the family (Kreisman & Joy, 1974; Hendersen et al., 1979; Hinchcliffe et al., 1975, 1977). This is engendered not merely by concern about current symptoms and handicaps, but also by the fear of future exacerbations. Because the manic-depressive patient may experience periods of euthymia or "normality," there is a tendency to view the disorder in the patient as having a somewhat benign course. Effective prophylactic medication, which controls and attenuates acute mood swings, tends to minimize mental health professionals' awareness of continuing distress associated with the disorder for the patient and family (Jamison, Gerner, & Goodwin, 1979). The malignant quality of manic-depressive illness is insufficiently appreciated. The functional impairment found among many bipolar patients in follow-up studies, and the havoc and disruption reported in their occupational, family, and social lives, suggests that, in spite of adequate drug treatment, disturbing problems persist for many, impeding the optimal emotional growth and development of both the patient and family members. Despite their significant effect on symptoms, lithium and other somatic therapies by themselves have little impact on interpersonal problems that may have developed in the course of the illness (Rounsaville, Prusoff, & Weisman, 1980).

Families of patients with depressive illnesses experience a wide range of difficulties (Keitner, Miller, Epstein, Bishop, & Fruzzetti, 1987; Coyne, 1976; Papolos & Papolos, 1992), yet few studies exist that have assessed the relationship of family functioning to course and outcome in patients with bipolar disorder or recurrent major depression. There is good reason to believe that factors other than compliance with medication, such as psychosocial stressors, affect the response to lithium salts, and, therefore, affect the subsequent clinical course and social adjustment in patients with recurrent mood disorders (Miklowitz, Goldstein, Nuachterlein, Snyder, & Mintz, 1988). Unfortunately, most studies that have attempted to identify environmental factors that influence the response to treatment have suffered from a number of methodological shortcomings, including small sample size, lack of control groups, diagnostically heterogeneous samples, assessments of only one family member, and lack of validated instruments to measure family functioning. A few studies are notable for their methodological rigor and testable conclusions (Miklowitz et al., 1988; Keitner et al., 1987). Miklowitz and colleagues applied methods that previously were effective in identifying psychosocial factors relevant to the course of other major psychiatric illnesses. This study used measures of family attitudes obtained from key relatives of recently hospitalized manic bipolar patients, including expressed emotion (EE) and interactional behaviors, affective style (AS), both of which have been found to predict relapse in schizophrenia (Vaughn, Snyder, Jones, Freeman, &

Falloon, 1984). In this study, levels of intrafamilial EE and AS were found to predict the likelihood of patient relapse in bipolar disorder as well, and the predictive relationship observed was independent of patient medication, baseline symptoms, demographics, and illness history.

Although findings from several studies of combined individual psychotherapy and pharmacotherapy of unipolar depression (Rounsaville et al., 1980; Frank & Kupfer, 1986) suggest that poor response to treatment and a greater likelihood of relapse are associated with marital and family conflict, few reported studies have been conducted that include an assessment of the family's understanding of or response to the illness as a variable that may influence treatment outcome. Keitner and colleagues (1987), in a well-controlled study designed to address concerns regarding the relationship between family functioning and depressive disorders, found that depressive episodes were significantly shorter (4.1 months) in those families that improved in family functioning during follow-up than in those that did not (8.1 months) improve.

Reports from an ongoing study (Frank & Kupfer, 1986) of a combined treatment approach to patients with recurrent mood disorders suggest that the addition of psychotherapy, as well as an educational workshop offered to patients and their families, may reduce the risk of relapse to a rate below 10%. If replicated, this finding would be of great clinical significance, since patients with recurrent depression ordinarily experience a 40% rate of relapse within four to five months following recovery from an acute episode (Prien et al., 1984). Unfortunately, existing studies have tended to assess single dimensions of family health or pathology, and no well-controlled studies have investigated the effects of family psychoeducational models, while there is strong evidence from schizophrenia research to indicate a rather robust effect of family psychoeducational approaches in the prevention of relapse and costly rehospitalization in the treatment of that major psychiatric disorder (Anderson, Hogarty, & Reiss, 1986).

While only a handful of studies have examined the questions whose answers might inform the development of an integrated treatment approach, it is incumbent on clinicians and mental health administrators to formulate more rational multidimensional treatment strategies anchored by the cumulative data provided by genetic, family, and outcome studies. Although the involvement of the family in the treatment process departs from rigidly held tenets of the traditional one-on-one doctor–patient relationship and raises issues of patient confidentiality, it is nevertheless recommended that the education of high-risk families be a cornerstone of any such treatment paradigm. The view that these multigenerational, familial recurrent illnesses have profound effects on relationships within the family, that earlier onset in the parental generation predisposes to earlier onset in the subsequent generation and predicts a much higher risk of illness in first-degree relatives, and that juvenile-onset affective disorder frequently goes unrecognized and undertreated (Joyce, 1984) should provide the impetus. A multigenerational perspective would necessarily lead clinicians and designers of mental health services to view family education as a primary goal for mental health policy.

THE FAMILY PSYCHOEDUCATIONAL APPROACH: AN INTEGRATED TREATMENT MODALITY

A model program to educate patients and family members was developed at the Albert Einstein College of Medicine/Montefiore Medical Center (Papolos & Moltz, 1984). It is based on Drs. Carol Anderson, Gerald Hogarty, and Douglas Reiss' psychoeducational work with schizophrenic patients and their families in Baltimore and Pittsburgh. The approach is a practical one that goes far, in a short time, toward clearing up the myths surrounding the illness. It seeks to increase the stability of the family environment by decreasing the family members' anxiety about the patient and increasing their self-confidence and knowledge about the disorder. It improves the family's capacity to react constructively to the patient during episodes of illness and addresses the heritable nature of the condition. The approach typically requires five patient and family meetings.

Description of the Psychoeducational Approach

If the first of the five sessions takes place following an initial episode, or if the family has not been involved in previous episodes, it is often the case that each member has some theory about the disorder. The goal of the first meeting, then, is to understand the family members' theories. They are asked to entertain a medical hypothesis about the cause of the disorder and are given information that describes in a question-and-answer format the nature, symptoms, and course of major affective disorders (Papolos, 1987).

The provision of information usually sparks a lively discussion among the family members and the psychiatrist in the second session. There are often emotional responses to the idea that the illness has a biological basis and is heritable. Questions about medication efficacy, side effects, and criteria for long-term maintenance are discussed also. In the meetings that follow, the patient is encouraged to describe his or her subjective experience of the symptoms and the limitations they impose, and the family members begin to pinpoint how they responded to the loss of the ill member during episodes of depression or mania. How did each person try to rouse the patient from his or her illness during episodes of depression? How did each family member attempt to set limits for the patient during episodes of mania? What feelings were aroused when the attempts failed?

During the fifth and final session, the therapist and the family review what has been learned: the nature, course, and treatment of the disorder; the effects on the relationship system; and the strategies developed to avoid the conflicts that arose as a consequence of the patient's change in behavior during an acute episode of illness. If all goes well, the conflict among family members is decreased, healthy coping skills are attained, and the family becomes more of a support for the patient.

The goals of the psychoeducational approach are as follows:

- To enable the patient and family to accept the idea that the patient has a medical disorder that may be recurrent and that produces symptoms that affect mood, self-esteem, thinking, speech, activity, sleep, appetite, and social and sexual behavior.
- To teach the patient and family to identify and label the specific symptoms that occur at the onset of an episode.
- To facilitate the acknowledgment that the most recent and/or past episodes have had an impact on the way family members view the

patient and to identify and describe any change in their attitudes toward the patient and in the pattern of their relationship with the patient during and after an episode of either mania or depression.
- To examine the changes that occur in the usual caretaking roles during an acute episode.
- To convey that major affective disorders are familial disorders and so may affect others in the family, and to provide information about studies that report the diagnostic difficulties frequently encountered with early-onset and first-time episodes.
- To explain the potential advantages and risks of preventive treatment, as well as of no treatment, from the time the acute episode is brought under control.
- To explain the importance of long term monitoring, including laboratory tests, and to encourage the family to share in the decision to initiate maintenance treatment.
- To teach the family to distinguish medication side effects from the symptoms of illness.

The following case illustrates a number of ways in which the psychoeducational approach worked for a patient and for her family members. It highlights the common finding of misdiagnosis as schizophrenia in adolescent-onset mania, and underscores the profound psychological impact of some of the common symptoms of mania when they are not viewed as occurring in the context of a medical disorder.

J.C. is a 27-year-old, single, white Catholic woman of Italian-American descent. At the age of 16, she had her first episode of hypomania, in which she became uncharacteristically and excessively sexual, propositioning family friends and passersby on the street. She also had symptoms of insomnia and pressured speech, and felt euphoric. This first episode ushered in a period of promiscuity and drug abuse.

Thinking that she was a "bad girl" who had disgraced the family, the patient's father reacted violently, and began to beat her for her sexual indiscretions. J.C. became more and more agitated and eventually required hospitalization. At the hospital, she was misdiagnosed as schizophrenic, treated with the antipsychotic drug, thioridazine and discharged several weeks after admission when her agitation had subsided.

The patient continued to suffer periodic exacerbations of her illness over the next six years. During the hypomanic episodes, her behavior bewildered the other members of her family since they assumed that she had received appropriate treatment and they did not attribute her excessive sexuality and argumentativeness to a medical disorder. Her father continued to lose his temper, to confine her to the home, and to beat her severely.

At the age of 22, following a second hospitalization, the diagnosis of bipolar affective disorder was established, and J.C. responded well to a trial of lithium. Her relationship with her parents eased somewhat, but they never fully understood the periodic nature of her disorder. The threat of physical violence loomed over the household, and yet the patient's parents feared that any confrontation or stress might trigger another episode.

Four years later, J.C.'s lithium level fell below the therapeutic range. She felt herself becoming ill and drove to the hospital, where she requested voluntary admission. She told the resident in the emergency room that she hadn't slept for a week and had racing thoughts and increased sexual feelings. Her speech was pressured and she was hypertalkative on admission. The dosage of lithium was increased and within a week she was free of symptoms.

The patient's psychiatrist felt that J.C. and her family could benefit from the psychoeducational approach and the social worker invited the family to participate in the five-session family therapy.

At the first family meeting, it became apparent that J.C. had a profound fear of her father as a consequence of the beatings she had suffered. Mr. C. expressed a desire to learn more about his daughter's illness, although initially he did not read the pamphlet on mood disorders that was given to him. When asked about his response to J.C.'s illness, he reported that he would typically stop talking to her when she appeared agitated, lest he set her off again. If the conversation became too heated, he used a hand gesture that prompted his wife and J.C. to stop talking. He felt that the only solution to the problem was to have his daughter move out of the house.

During the family sessions, Mr. C. reported how guilty he felt over the way he had treated his daughter. He admitted that the guilt and the outrage at his daughter's behavior left him feeling helpless. Mrs. C. appeared to be a quiet, passive mother and wife who possessed a greater tolerance of and sympathy for her daughter's behavior, but who would support her husband's viewpoint at all costs.

During the five sessions, the nature of J.C.'s periodic disorder was explained to the family. The psychiatrist clarified that J.C.'s hypersexual behavior was a symptom of the illness and not the volitional act of a "bad child." This led the family to the realization that she had been punished and shunned for behavior that was out of her control. Mr. C. apologized for the years of physical abuse, and the family elected to continue in twice-monthly family treatment to further work through their responses to J.C.'s illness.

When a relative experiences recurrent episodes of depression or mania, there is a disruptive and disorganizing effect on family life. The other members of the family are faced with the challenge of looking after and providing for the needs of their relative—often in an atmosphere of confusion, isolation, embarrassment, anger, and guilt. Before long, the individual needs of all the family members are ignored as each tries to grapple with the tension that accompanies these disorders. The following case points to the generational impact of these conditions, and the usefulness in framing the treatment process within the family group.

E.G. began to suffer serious periods of hypomania and depression during his college years. Despite these interruptions, he persevered, graduated from college, and found meaningful work. Although his episodes had been muted by drugs, he continued to have mood swings. These periodic episodes of hypomania and depression flew in the face of his attempts to establish himself independently of his parents and so he continued to live at home. He was encouraged by his parents after each setback, but he felt a growing sense of isolation and a loss of credibility in the aftermath of each episode. He was having a great deal of difficulty understanding and coping with his family's reaction to his illness. The patient's mother appeared nervous around him and was overly sensitive to any changes in his mood. His father, a physician, denied that his son's problems were really serious, and his younger brother, once his closest confidant, refused to be seen with him or to invite friends to their home.

E.G. and his family came for consultation initially with questions about the medical treatment—his expectation and that of his family was that he should no longer have mood swings. The fact that he continued to have brief periods of depression and hypomania was unacceptable and meant to them that something was wrong with the way in which his treatment was being managed. Moreover, he was having trouble with a lithium tremor. It was a source of embarrassment to his family and he was increasingly sensing that his mood and behavior were a focus of concern in the household. He felt under constant pressure to explain even minor changes in his moods.

Fearing that the least stress might set off another episode, the family had been living with a prolonged uncertainty and apprehensiveness. In such an atmosphere, E.G.'s behavior and natural expression of such emotions as joy, sadness, and anger came under close scrutiny, and even suspicion. The family, in the position of being an early-warning system of impending mood swings, had stepped into the role of prosecuting attorney: The patient was faced with seemingly endless questions and doubts and was asked to provide motives for almost every act. This was a corrosive atmosphere for everyone concerned. The patient's credibility and competence as a person were called into question by the often unspoken suspicions of his motives and emotions and the family was placed under a terrible strain.

The effect of these constant unspoken suspicions had robbed the patient of his sense of credibility, which eventually can become crippling to self-esteem. Paradoxically, this atmosphere of mistrust within such a family springs not from prejudice, but from a natural inclination to care about and to protect the person who is ill. But the quality of the caring can be derailed by fear, denial, and lack of knowledge. Constant sympathetic attempts to raise a person's spirits during a depression are often of no avail, and family members feel frustrated, and then resentful or angry and despairing as they sense that no matter what they do, it does not make a difference.

A number of things changed as a result of the family sessions. By learning more specifically about the nature of E.G.'s condition and the natural course of the illness, the family members were able to begin to work collaboratively rather than at cross-purposes. E.G.'s mother learned that her desire to protect her son from any further episodes by scrutinizing his every change in mood was creating an unbearable tension in the household, sapping her energy and needlessly alienating her son. She lessened the demands on E.G. and her own unrealistic expectations of what treatment could accomplish.

E.G.'s physician father at first had a great deal of difficulty with acknowledging the emotional impact of his son's condition. He had chosen to minimize and downplay his son's symptoms, saying that he thought it best to reassure him rather than to offer him sympathy. He initially spoke about the cost of psychiatric treatment and focused his anger on the discriminatory policies of his firm's insurance coverage. However, he was unwilling to rock the boat and to appeal a decision that limited reimbursement.

Not long into the family sessions, E.G.'s father acknowledged that he, too, had experienced numerous episodes of depression, but without seeking treatment; he had chosen to "tough it out." As he spoke in more depth about his own experiences with depression, he confided a secret that had been kept from his family for years. His own father had been diagnosed as manic-depressive and had committed suicide. E.G.'s father had been unable to face the idea that there was some association between his own depressions, the suicide of his father, and his son's condition. The anger he harbored toward his father and the shame that had forced him to conceal his own pain had surfaced in subtle and self-destructive ways. As a result of the family treatment, he came to realize that the denial of his illness had contributed to the double messages he communicated to his son—on the one hand, minimizing his symptoms, and on the other hand, expecting him to be able to control his mood swings voluntarily. Denial, fear, and shame had cast long shadows—from grandfather to father to son.

These powerful forces can immobilize the most caring of families. And with a heritable illness such as manic-depression, far more than the genetic vulnerability can span the generations.

After learning about and accepting the biological basis of the condition and its heritability within his own family, E.G's father was, for the first time, able to seek treatment for himself and to empathize with his son's struggle. Previously, he had been shackled by a sense of shame and the fear that he would be viewed contemptuously in his work and social circles. Now, he felt empowered by his new perspective as to the medical basis of the condition.

Our experience in applying the family psychoeducational approach with over 400 families of diverse ethnic and social backgrounds has reified our view that these conditions must be seen within the larger context of the multigenerational family, and that family members can serve as potent allies in the prevention of relapse.

GENETIC COUNSELING: AN EXTENSION OF THE PSYCHOEDUCATIONAL APPROACH

Once families learn and accept that mood disorders are heritable, some become interested in exploring the degree of risk in more depth. Many professionals in the health sciences have long felt that psychiatric disorders are not a fit subject for genetic counseling because of their unknown etiology. If we are not sure what gene defects are involved in psychiatric disorders, how can we estimate risks with any certainty? Indeed, knowing that there is a genetic basis for a disease is no substitute for understanding how the genetic mechanism works. However, some physical diseases with etiologies no more certain than those of most psychiatric disorders are commonly the subjects of genetic counseling and education. Such problems make counseling more difficult, but they do not preclude it.

Psychiatrists have recourse to other practical means for estimating the risk of recurrence for ambiguously inherited disorders. Great advances have been made during recent years and ingenious methods have been developed for examining the interaction between heredity and environmental factors. At the simplest level, investigators have used the "proband method," in which an index case with a particular diagnosis (e.g., bipolar disorder) is identified, and rates of illness in members of the subject's family are compared with rates in some appropriate comparison group (e.g., relatives of individuals who have never been psychiatrically ill). Many such large-scale epidemiologic studies have resulted in pools of data that allow psychiatrists to make reasonably accurate empirical risk estimates.

Although the relative contribution of genetic factors is not precisely known, it is possible to determine the empirical risk for the development of illness in relatives of ill patients. In Chapter 8, Dr. Shalom Feinberg describes the experience in a homogeneous community, the Orthodox Jewish community, and underscores basic principles of genetic counseling derived from his clinical experience.

REFERENCES

Akiskal, H., Downs, J., Parri, J., Jordan, P., Watson, S., Dougherty, D., & Pruitt, D. B. (1985). Affective disorders in referred children and younger siblings of manic-depressives. *Archives of General Psychiatry, 42,* 996–1003.

Anderson, C. M., Hogarty, G. F., & Reiss, D. J. (1986). Family treatment of schizophrenic patients: A psychoeducational approach. *Schizophrenia Bulletin,* 490–582.

Angst, J., Weis, P., Grof, P., Baastrup, P. C., & Schou, M. (1970). Lithium prophylaxis in recurrent affective disorders. *British Journal of Psychiatry, 116,* 604–614.

Baastrup, P. C., & Schou, M. (1967). Lithium as a prophylactic agent. Its effectiveness against recurrent depressions and manic-depressive psychosis. *Archives of General Psychiatry, 16,* 162–172.

Baldessarini, R. J. (1983). *Biomedical aspects of depression and its treatment.* Washington, DC: American Psychiatric Press.

Baldessarini, R. J., & Tohen, M. (1988). Is there a long-term protective effect of mood-altering agents in unipolar depressive disorder? *In Current trends.* Berlin, Heidelberg: Springer-Verlago.

Beardslee, W. R., Bemporad, J., Keller, M. B., & Klerman, G. L. (1983). Children of parents with major affective disorders: A review. *American Journal of Psychiatry, 140,* 825–832.

Beardslee, W. R., Keller, M. B., & Klerman, G. L. (1985). Children of parents with affective disorder. *International Journal of Family Psychiatry, 6,* 283–299.

Bertelsen, A., Harvald, B., & Hauge, M. (1977). Danish twin study of manic-depressive disorders. *British Journal of Psychiatry, 130,* 330–351.

Boyd, J. H., & Weissman, M. M. (1981). Epidemiology of affective disorders: A reexamination and future directions. *Archives of General Psychiatry, 38,* 1039–1046.

Brody, G. H., & Forehand, R. (1986). Maternal perceptions of child maladjustment as a function of the combined influence of child behavior and maternal depression. *Journal of Consulting Clinical Psychology, 54,* 237–240.

Brown, G. W., Birley, J. L. T., & Wing J. K. (1972). Influence of family life on the course of schizophrenic disorders: A replication. *British Journal of Psychiatry, 121,* 241–258.

Carter, A. S., Pauls, D. C., & Egeland, J. A. (1992). Differential risk for affective disorders among the Old Order Amish: An examination of the influence of maternal and paternal diagnostic status.

Cochran, S. D. (1984). Preventing medical noncompliance in the outpatient treatment of bipolar disorder. *Journal of Consulting Clinical Psychology, 52,* 873–878.

Coryell, W., Andreasen, N. C., Endicott, J., & Keller, M. (1987). The significance of past manic or hypomanic in the course and outcome of manic-depression. *American Journal of Psychiatry, 144,* 309–315.

Coyne, J. C. (1976). Depression and the response of others. *Journal of Abnormal Psychology, 85,* 186–193.

Davenport, Y. B., Adland, M. L., Gold, P. W., & Goodwin, F. K. (1979). Psychodynamic features of multigenerational families. *American Journal of Orthopsychiatry, 49,* 24–35.

Davenport, Y. B., Zahn-Waxler, C., Adland, M. L., & Mayfield, A. (1983). Early child-rearing practices in families with a manic-depressive parent. *American Journal of Psychiatry, 140,* 230–238.

Decina, P., Kestenbaum, C. J., Farber, S., Kron, L., Gargan, M., Sackeim, H. A., & Fieve, R. R. (1983). Clinical and psychological assessment of children of bipolar probands. *American Journal of Psychiatry, 140,* 548–553.

Dunner, D. L. (1986). Recent genetic studies of bipolar and unipolar affective disorders. In J. T. Coyne (Ed.), *Essential papers in depression* (pp. 449–458). New York: New York University Press.

Faraone, S. V., Kremen, W. S., & Tsuang, M. T. (1990). Genetic transmission of major affective disorders: Quantitative models and linkage analysis. *Psychological Bulletin, 108,* 109–127.

Frank, E., & Kupfer, D. (1986). Psychotherapeutic approaches to the treatment of recurrent unipolar depression: Work in progress. *Psychopharmacology Bulletin, 22,* 558–563.

Frank, E., Kupfer, D. J., Perel, J. M., Cones, C., Jarrett, D. B., Mallinger, A. G., Thase, M. E., McEachran, A. B., & Grochweinski, V. J. (1990). Three year outcomes for maintenance therapies in recurrent depression. *Archives of General Psychiatry, 47,* 1093–1099.

Gershon, E. S., McKnew, D., Cytryn, L., Hamovit, J., Schreiber, J., Hibbs, E., & Pellegrini, D. (1985). Diagnosis in school-age children of bipolar affective disorder patients and normal controls. *Journal of Affective Disorders 8,* 283–291.

Gershon, E. S., Berrettini, W., Nurnberger, J., Jr., & Goldin, L. R. (1987a). Genetics of affective illness. In H. Y. Meltzer (Ed.), *Psychopharmacology: The third generation of progress* (pp. 481-491), New York: Raven.

Gershon, E. S., Hamovit, J. H., Guroff, J. J. & Nurnberger, H. (1987b). Birth-cohort changes in manic and depressive disorders in relatives of bipolar and schizoaffective patients. *Archives of General Psychiatry, 44*, 314-319.

Goodwin, F. K. (1989). The biology of recurrence: New directions for the pharmacologic bridge. *Journal of Clinical Psychiatry, 50*, (12 suppl.) 40-44.

Grigoroiu-Serbanescu, M., Christodorescu, D., Jipescu, I., Totoescu, A., Marinescu, E., & Ardlean, V. (1989). Psychopathology in children aged 10-17 of bipolar parents: Psychopathology rate and correlates of the severity of the psychopathology. *Journal of Affective Disorders, 16*, 167-179.

Hammen, C., Burge, D., Burney, E., & Adrian, C. (1990). Longitudinal study of diagnoses in children of women with unipolar and bipolar affective disorder. *Archives of General Psychiatry, 47*, 1112-1117.

Hammen, C., Gordon, D., Burge, D., Adrian, C., Jaenicke, C., & Hiroto, D. (1987a). Children of depressed mothers: Maternal strain and symptom predictors of dysfunction. *Journal of Abnormal Psychology, 96*, 190-198.

Hammen, C., Gordon, D., Burge, D., Adrian, C., Jaenicke, C., & Hiroto, D. (1987b). Maternal affective disorders, illness and stress. Risk for children's psychopathology. *American Journal of Psychiatry, 144*, 736-740.

Hatfield, A. B. (1979). The family as a partner in the treatment of mental illness. *Hospital and community psychiatry, 30* (5), 338-340.

Hendersen, S. (1979). The patients primary group. *British Journal of Psychiatry, 132*, 74-86.

Hinchcliffe, M., Hooper, D., Roberts, E. J., & Vaughan, P. W. (1975). A study of the interactions between depressed patients and their spouses. *British Journal of Psychiatry, 126*, 164-172.

Hinchcliffe, M., Hooper, D., Roberts, E. J., & Vaughan, P. W. (1977). The melancholy marriage: An inquiry into the interaction of depression. II. Expressiveness. *British Journal of Medical Psychology, 50*, 125-142.

Jamison, K. R., & Akiskal, H. S. (1983). Medication compliance in patients with bipolar disorder. *Psychiatric Clinics of North America, 6*, 175-192.

Jamison, K. R., Gerner, R. H., Goodwin, F. K. (1979). Patient and physician attitudes toward lithium. *Archives of General Psychiatry, 36*, 866-869.

Joyce, P. R. (1984). Age of onset in bipolar affective disorder and misdiagnosis as schizophrenia. *Psychological Medicine, 14,* 145–149.

Keisling, R. (1981). Underdiagnosis of manic-depressive illness in a hospital unit. *American Journal of Psychiatry, 138,* 5.

Keitner, G. I., Miller, I. W., Epstein, N. B., Bishop, D. S., & Fruzzetti, A. E. (1987). Family functioning and the course of major depression. Comp. Psychiatry Jan-Feb: *28* (1), 54–64.

Keller, M. B., Klerman, G. L., Lavori, P. W., Fawcett, J. A., Coryell, W., Andreasen, N. C., & Endicott, J. (1982). Treatment received by depressed patients. *Journal of the American Medical Association, 248,* 1841–1855.

Keller, M. B., Lavori, P. W., Rice, J., Coryell, W., & Hirschfeld, R. M. (1986). The persistent risk of chronicity in recurrent episodes of nonbipolar major depressive disorder: A prospective follow-up. *American Journal of Psychiatry, 143,* 24–28.

Kety, S. S., Rosenthal, D., Wender, P. H., et al. (1968). The types and prevalence of mental illness in the biological and adoptive families of adopted schizophrenics. In D. Rosenthal & S. S. Kety (Eds.), *The transmission of schizophrenia* (pp. 345–362). Oxford, England: Pergamon.

Klerman, G. L., Lavori, P. W., Rice, J., Reich, T., Endicott, J., Andreasen, N. C., Keller, M. B., & Hirschfeld, R. M. A. (1985). Birth-cohort trends in rates of major depressive disorder among relatives of patients with affective disorder. *Archives of General Psychiatry, 42,* 689–693.

Kochanska, G., Radke-Yarrow, M., Kuczynske, L., Friedman, S. L. (1987). Normal and affectively ill mothers' beliefs about their children. *American Journal of Orthopsychiatry, 57,* 345–350.

Kreisman, D. E., & Joy, V. D. (1974). Family response to the mental illness of a relative: A review of the literature. *Schizophrenia Bulletin, 1* (10), 34–57.

Kukopulos, A., & Reginaldi, D. (1980). Recurrences of manic-depressive episodes during lithium treatment. In M. Schou (Ed.), *Handbook of lithium therapy.* Lancaster, PA: MTP Press.

Kukopulos, A., Reginaldi, D., Laddomada, P., Floris, G., Serra, G., & Tondo, L. (1980). Course of the manic-depressive cycle and changes caused by treatments. *Pharmakopsychiatrie Neuro-Psychopharmakologie, 13,* 156–167.

Landolt, A. D. (1957). Follow-up studies on circular manic-depressive reactions occurring in the young. *Bulletin of the New York Academy of Medicine, 33,* 65–73.

LaRoche, C., Scheiner, R., Lester, E. P., Benieralcis, C., & Marrache, M. (1987). Children of parents with manic-depressive illness: A follow-up study. *Canadian Journal of Psychiatry, 32,* 563–569.

Leonhard, K., Berman, R., & Robins, E. (Eds.), *Aufteilung der Endogenen Psychosen (The classification of endogenous psychoses)* (5th ed.). New York: Irvington.

Maj, M., Raffaele, P., & Starace, F. (1989). Previous pattern of course of illness as a prediction of response to lithium prophylaxis in bipolar patients. *Journal of Disorders, 17,* 237–241.

Mendlewicz, J., & Rainer, J. (1977). Adoption study supporting genetic transmission in manic-depressive illness. *Nature, 268,* 327–329.

Merinkangas, K. R., Prusoff, B. A., Kupfer, D. J., & Frank, E. (1985). Marital adjustment in major depression. *Journal of Affective Disorders, 1,* 5–11.

Miklowitz, D. J., Goldstein, M. J., Nuechterlein, K. H., Snyder, K. S., & Mintz, J. (1988). Family factors and the course of bipolar affective disorder. *Archives of General Psychiatry, 45,* 225–231.

Olsen, T. (1961). Follow-up study of manic-depressive patients whose first attack occurred before the age of 19. *Acta Psychiatrica Scandanavica, 162* (suppl.) 45–51.

Papolos, D. F. (1987). Mood disorders: Depression and manic-depression. NAMI Medical Information Series. National Alliance for the Mentally Ill, Alexandria, VA.

Papolos, D. F., & Moltz, D. (1984). The psychoeducational approach to major affective disorders. Presentation at the American Family Therapy Association, New York.

Papolos, D. F., & Papolos, J. D. (1992). *Overcoming depression (rev. ed.).* New York: Harper Collins.

Perris, C. (1966). A study of bipolar (manic-depressive) and unipolar recurrent depressive psychoses. *Acta Psychiatrica Scandanavica, 42* (suppl.), 194.

Pope, H. G., & Lipinski, J. F., Jr. (1983). Diagnosis in schizophrenia and manic-depressive illness: A reassessment of the specificity of schizophrenic symptoms in light of current research. *Archives of General Psychiatry, 35,* 811–822.

Post, R. M., & Weiss, S. R. B. (1989). Sensitization, kindling and anticonvulsants in mania. *Journal of Clinical Psychiatry, 50* (12 suppl.), 23–30.

Prien, R. F., & Kupfer, D. J. (1986). Combination drug therapy for major depressive episodes: How long should it be maintained? *American Journal of Psychiatry, 143,* 18–23.

Prien, R. F., Kupfer, D. J., Mansky, P. A., Small, J. G., Tauson, V. B., Voss, C. B., & Johnson, W. E. (1984). Drug therapy in the prevention of recurrences in unipolar and bipolar affective disorders: Report of the NIMH Collaborative Study Group comparing lithium carbonate, imipramine, and a lithium carbonate-imipramine combination. *Archives of General Psychiatry, 41,* 1096–1104.

Rice, J. P., Reich, T., Andreasen, N. C., Endicott, J., van Eerdewegh, M., Fishman, R., Hirschfeld, R. M. A., & Klerman, G. L. (1987). The familial transmission of bipolar illness. *Archives of General Psychiatry, 44,* 441–447.

Rounsaville, B. J., Prusoff, B. A., & Weissman, M. M. (1980). The course of marital disputes in depressed women: A 48-month follow-up study. *Comprehensive Psychiatry, 21,* 111–118.

Schou, M. (1979). Lithium as a prophylactic agent in unipolar affective illness: Comparison with cyclic antidepressants. *Archives of General Psychiatry, 36,* 849–851.

Stancer, H. C., Persad, E., Wagener, D. K., & Jorna, T. (1987). Evidence for homogeneity of major depression and bipolar affective disorder. *Journal of Psychiatric Research, 21* (1), 37–53.

Strober, M., & Carlson, G. (1982). Bipolar illness in adolescents with major depression: Clinical, genetic, and psychopharmacologic predictors in a three- to four-year prospective follow-up investigation. *Archives of General Psychiatry, 39,* 549–555.

Strober, M., Morrell, W., Burroughs, J., Lampert, C., Danforth, H., & Freeman, R. (1988). A family study of bipolar I disorder in adolescence: Early onset of symptoms linked to increased familial loading and lithium resistance. *Journal of Affective Disorders, 15,* 255–268.

Tsuang, M. T., & Faraone, S. V. (1990). *The genetics of mood disorders.* Baltimore, MD: Johns Hopkins University.

Tsuang, M. T., & Vandermey, R. (1980). *Genes and the mind.* London, England: Oxford University Press.

Vaughn, C. E., Snyder, K. S., Jones, S., Freeman, W. B., & Falloon, I. R. H. (1984). Family factors in schizophrenic relapse: Replication in California of British research on expressed emotion. *Archives of General Psychiatry, 41,* 1169–1177.

Weissman, M. M., Gammon, G. D., & John, K. (1987). Children of depressed parents. *Archives of General Psychiatry. 44,* 847–853.

Weissman, M. M, Prusoff, B. A., Gammon, G. D., et al. (1984). *Journal of the American Academy of Child Psychiatry, 23,* 78–84.

Weissman, M. M., Warner, V., Wickramaratne, P., & Prusoff, B. A. (1988). Early onset major depression in patients and their children. *Journal of Affective Disorders, 15,* 269–277.

Welner, A., Welner, Z., & Fishman, R. (1979). Psychiatric adolescent in patients: Eight- to ten-year follow-up. *Archives of General Psychiatry, 36,* 635–643.

Wender, P. H., Kety, S. S., Rosenthal, D., Schulsinger, F., Ortmann, J., & Lunde, I. (1986). Psychiatric disorders in the biological and adoptive families of adopted individuals with affective disorders. *Archives of General Psychiatry, 43,* 923–929.

Zahn-Waxler, C., Cummings, E. M., & McKnew, D. H. (1984). Young offspring of depressed parents: A population at risk for affective problems. In D. Cichetti & K. Schneider-Rosen (Eds.), *Childhood depression: New directions for child development series no. 26* (pp. 81–105). San Francisco, CA: Jossey-Bass.

Zis, A. P., & Goodwin, F. K. (1979). Major affective disorder as a recurrent illness. *Archives of General Psychiatry, 36* (8 Spec. No.) 835–839.

8

Genetic Counseling Issues in Affective Disorders
The Orthodox Jewish Community

SHALOM FEINBERG

While research questions delving into the genetic aspects of mood disorders have become more complex and the methodology more sophisticated, the concerns of patients and their families about genetic predisposition and heritability continue to raise strong emotional issues. The range of concerns is articulated by such questions as: "Is this inherited?" "Are my children at risk?" "Should I marry into this family?" Clinicians need a working knowledge of psychiatric genetics in general, and of affective illness in particular, so that they can be properly equipped to address these issues (Pardes, Kaufmann, Pincus, & West, 1989). The possibility that one has a *genetic* illness may conjure up for some the mistaken, anxiety-provoking image of an inevitable, incurable disease (Tsuang, 1978). Psychiatric genetic counseling can supply information, help alleviate anxiety and guilt, and assist individuals in formulating personal plans. It forms an essential component of the psychoeducational approach described in Chapter 7.

This chapter examines these issues from the perspective of one specific cultural subgroup, the Orthodox Jewish community. From our genetic counseling work with this community, we have gained valuable information that enriches our understanding of the psychiatric genetic counseling process. We describe relevant features of this community, offer an overview of the genetics of affective illness, and relate it to the counseling process.

THE ORTHODOX JEWISH COMMUNITY

The Jewish community is actually composed of multiple subgroups differing in cultural origins, as well as in levels of religious commitment and practice. Orthodox Jews, the smallest segment of Judaism, are characterized by their staunch belief in God and strict observance and practice of the *halacha*, the Jewish law as passed down over the generations (Liebman, 1983). Relevant for this discussion, the Orthodox Jewish community has also been distinguished throughout the centuries by a very low rate of intermarriage, a relatively low incidence of alcohol and substance abuse (Glassner & Berg, 1984; Feinberg & Feinberg, 1985), and the great importance placed on immersing oneself in the study and mastery of the Torah and the Talmud.

Marriage and procreation are among the most important tenets of Judaism, and fulfillment of these biblical commands is an extremely important priority for Orthodox Jews (Feldman, 1974). In view of the biblical mandate to "be fruitful and multiply," contraception and other means of birth control are unacceptable, especially among the ultraorthodox (Goshen-Gottstein, 1987). Securing the "right" marriage or *shiddach* for oneself or one's child—that is, procuring a prestigious mate, or one who originates from a prestigious family—is also a tradition dating back to biblical times. It is viewed as a means of best fulfilling these commands and perpetuating the Jewish heritage through one's family. The Orthodox community has very fluid lines of communication through which to obtain information about a potential marital partner despite being geographically dispersed around the world.

Though there is much concern in the general population about being labeled psychiatrically ill, there appears to be even greater concern in the Orthodox Jewish community. Despite reports of the increased use of mental heath services by Orthodox Jews (Wikler, 1979), unmet mental health needs persist. Both Orthodox mental health professionals and Orthodox rabbis have reported that the potential stigma associated with the acknowledgment of the need for treatment of psychiatric problems and the request for such treatment is a primary cause of these needs being unmet (Feinberg & Feinberg, 1985, 1986).

In large measure, this problem relates to what has been called "shiddach anxiety" (Levitz, 1979; Feinberg, 1989). This term refers to the fear that features of one's family will be viewed negatively by others in the consideration of a family member for a potential marriage, or shiddach, thereby damaging one's chances for a more prestigious marriage or dashing hopes of marriage altogether. This fear is particularly intense when the family feature is related to mental illness (Feinberg & Feinberg, 1985; Goshen-Gottstein, 1987). This relates, in part, to the fact that Jews, as "People of the Book," place a high priority on intellectual and mental functioning (Grunblatt, 1985). Since psychiatric illness affects the mind and its ability to function, it directly threatens these values. Out of fear of stigmatizing one's family, one may not seek out mental health services until the situation is desperate and the problems more severe and more difficult to treat (Levitz, 1979; Feinberg & Feinberg, 1987).

Within Orthodox Jewry, there are subgroups along a wide spectrum of values, practices, and customs, ranging from the distinctly garbed Hasidic sects to the "modern Orthodox," who attempt to live in both secular and religious worlds. There is also variability along this continuum as to the intensity of concerns about stigmatization, as well as to how frequently mental health services are sought out when needed. For example, families closer to the so-called "right" of the Orthodox spectrum, including the Hasidic community, are generally more fearful of being stigmatized, and, therefore, are less accepting of psychiatric assistance (Feinberg & Feinberg, 1985).

GENETICS OF MOOD DISORDERS

Mode of Inheritance

Understanding the mode of the genetic transmission of affective disorders is an important aspect of arriving at an accurate prediction of risk within a family. Ideally, genetic-risk figures are based on empirical risk figures derived from family studies, the complete family history of the person or persons being counseled, and the mode of inheritance of illness within the specific family pedigree (Tsuang & Faraone, 1990). Unfortunately, research on the genetic transmission of affective illness has not produced consistent findings. There are reports of X-chromosome transmission (Baron et al., 1987), and autosomal dominant transmission that involved different chromosomes (e.g., Turner & King, 1983; Egeland et al., 1987), and lack of replication and confirmation of these single-locus modes of transmission (Berrettini et al., 1990; Campbell et al., 1984; Detera-Waldleigh et al., 1987; Kelsoe et al., 1989; Leckman, Gershon, McGuinniss, Targum, & Dibble, 1979), as well as inconclusive reports involving multifactorial-polygenic models (Slater & Tsuang, 1968; Morton & Maclean, 1974; Tsuang & Faraone, 1990). Taken together, these findings support the belief that there is heterogeneity in affective illness (Pardes et al., 1989; Tsuang & Faraone, 1990). In all likelihood, there are multiple potential modes of transmission. And not only may there be different modes of genetic transmission between families, but even within a single family. In large measure, this is probably due to the high frequency of assortative mating—the tendency of temperamentally similar individuals to marry—commonly noted in affected families.

Based on our present state of knowledge, a psychiatric genetic counselor is only rarely able to ascertain a given family's mode of inheritance of affective illness. For example, a family pedigree lacking father-to-son transmission with an excess of affected females suggests X-chromosome linkage (Baron, 1991a). However, to reach such a conclusion about the mode of transmission, one needs to assess a pedigree of adequate size. In an era of small, mobile families, this has proved problematic for counselors throughout the field of medical genetics (Skinner, 1990). Ascertaining for the presence of the X-linked form of bipolar disorder may become more important if preliminary evidence that suggests that this represents a more severe form of the disease is borne out (Baron, 1991a).

Incomplete Penetrance

There is a lack of complete penetrance for affective disorders. Penetrance is the probability that one possessing a specific genotype will express that trait. While it is far from clear what leads to incomplete penetrance, it clearly complicates risk prediction. For example, Egeland and colleagues (1987) found a maximum rate of penetrance for affective illness of 63% in their Amish studies. This implies that even if one could accurately identify those individuals who possess the ill genotype, only two thirds will actually manifest affective illness. However, it is not currently possible to predict which specific individuals with the ill genotype will express the illness.

Bipolar Spectrum

While it has been found that a bipolar proband increases the risk for the development of both unipolar and bipolar illness, unipolar disorder has not been convincingly shown to increase the risk for bipolar illness in other family members (Tsuang & Faraone, 1990). Unipolar illness within families that manifest bipolar illness may reflect the heterogeneity of expression of bipolar illness or cases where mania or hypomania has not yet become manifest. For example, Akiskal (1983) has described that many patients with "recurrent" unipolar depression have family histories of bipolar illness, and includes them in the "bipolar spectrum." Concepts such as the bipolar spectrum, the "soft" bipolar spectrum (Akiskal & Mallya, 1987), and affective spectrum disorders (Hudson & Pope, 1990) reflect the growing appreciation that bipolar illness in particular, and affective illness in general, may present in a variety of ways with different levels of overt psychopathology. These bipolar-related conditions include all major and minor affective disorders, schizoaffective disorder, eating disorders, panic disorder, and obsessive-compulsive disorder (Hudson & Pope 1990), as well as perhaps attention-deficit disorder (Biederman, Faraone, Keenan, & Tsuang, 1991). This information needs to be considered during the assessment and counseling process.

Empirical Risk Data

In terms of empirical risk data, the likelihood of developing a mood disorder, bipolar or unipolar, is many times greater in relatives of patients with mood disorders than in the general population (Gershon et al., 1982; Tsuang & Faraone, 1990). Similarly, the more heavily loaded a pedigree is for affective illness, the greater is the risk to unaffected relatives who have not passed the age of risk (Targum & Gershon, 1980). Additionally, in a family in which the incidence of a specific form of affective illness is high, such as bipolar II disorder, other family members may be at greater risk for that specific form of illness (Andreasen et al., 1987).

The genetic risk increases the closer within the pedigree one is to an individual diagnosed as having a mood disorder (Tsuang & Faraone, 1990). For example, as noted in Table 8–1, monozygotic twins, with 100% of their genes in common, have a higher concordance rate than dizygotic twins, who possess only 50% of their genes in common. This holds true for both bipolar and unipolar disorders. The concordance rate for monozygotic twins is approximately 75% for bipolar illness and 50% for unipolar illness (Schlesser & Altshuler, 1983; Gershon, 1990). This high rate of concordance appears to hold true even if the twins were reared apart (Price, 1968). In comparison, the risk to a twin of a dizygotic proband is almost the same as to that of other siblings, which is not greater than 15% to 25% (Gershon, 1990).

Overall, Baron (1991a) has noted a 13% to 35% risk of developing an affective illness of any type in a first-degree relative (parents, siblings, and offspring) of a bipolar patient. A unipolar patient offers a 10–20% risk to first-degree relatives for a unipolar disorder (Schlesser & Altshuler, 1983). The offspring of two affectively ill parents have at least double the risk for affective illness in comparison with the offspring of one affected parent (Gershon et al., 1982; Targum, 1988). Likewise, it has been consistently reported that the risk for an

TABLE 8–1
Estimated Morbidity Risk for Affective Illness in
Relatives of Bipolar and Unipolar Patients*

Relative	Bipolar Proband (%)	Unipolar Proband (%)
Monozygotic twin	75	50
Dizygotic twin	15–25	15–20
Offspring of one ill parent	15–30	15–20
Offspring of two ill parents	50–75	40–50
Sibling	15–25	10–20
Second-degree relative	3–7	3–5
Parent	15–20	10–15
General population	1	4

* Estimates for relatives of bipolar patients reflect the potential to develop unipolar, bipolar, and other spectrum disorders, whereas the relatives of unipolar patients primarily develop unipolar illness.

individual to develop affective illness significantly increases if both a parent and a sibling are ill, in contrast to an individual with either an affectively ill parent *or* sibling (Tsuang & Faraone, 1990). Estimates of the empirical risk to various relatives are offered in Table 8–1 as a general guide. It is important to note, however, that there is considerable variation in reported risk figures among investigators as a result of differences in methodology and diagnostic criteria.

While it has been estimated that second-degree relatives have a slightly greater risk for mood disorders than the general population (Targum, 1988), recent studies have suggested that the risk to second-degree relatives is similar to that of the general population for unipolar illness (Gershon et al., 1982; Tsuang & Faraone, 1990). Only bipolar probands increase the risk for mood disorder among their second-degree relatives, and only for bipolar, not unipolar, disorders. This is in concert with the preponderance of evidence that bipolar disorders have a greater genetic component than do unipolar disorders (Tsuang & Faraone, 1990). The propensity to develop the signs and symptoms of unipolar illness appears to be far more greatly influenced by nonfamilial environmental factors than bipolar disorder, and, therefore, produces a larger diverse group of phenocopies (nongenetic forms of the illness). Accordingly, it has been reported that the families of bipolar probands have twice as much affective illness as families with unipolar probands (Targum & Schulz, 1982). Moreover, 80 to 90% of bipolar patients will have a first-degree family member who suffers from some form of mood disorder (Schlesser & Altshuler, 1983).

Gender and Age of Onset

Females clearly appear to be at greater risk for unipolar illnesses than males, but they are equally at risk as males for bipolar illness (Weissman et al., 1988). As noted above, bipolar illness is transmitted less frequently from father to son than from mother to son, though this is not a consistent finding (Baron, 1991a). The risk of a same-sex sibling developing a mood disorder is greater than for a sibling of the opposite sex (Tsuang & Faraone, 1990).

An earlier age of onset of affective illness within a family member (in general, before the age of 40) increases the risk for all types of mood disorders among relatives, regardless of the sex of the proband or the relative (Rice et al., 1987; Tsuang & Faraone, 1990). Additionally, there appears to be a particularly strong hereditary component in adolescent-onset affective illness. For example, a recent report indicated that the occurrence of the onset of bipolar disorders during adolescence is associated with a rate of mood disorders or at any psychiatric illness in first-degree relatives of 33% and 58% respectively (Kutcher & Marton, 1991). In this study, adolescent-onset unipolar depression carried a lesser but likewise significant risk for first-degree relatives of 25% for a mood disorder and 47% for any psychiatric disorder. As many of the proband's siblings were quite young at the time the results of this study were reported and had not passed through the period of risk for illness, it is likely that these rates of risk will increase significantly over time.

Pharmacogenetics

There are a few studies that suggest that response to specific medications, such as lithium carbonate or antidepressants, may be genetically related (Angst, 1961; Pare & Mack, 1971; Mendlewicz, Fieve, & Stallone, 1973). That is, the response of one ill family member may predict a similar response by others in the family with psychiatric illness. However, other investigators have not observed such a relationship (Nurnberger, 1987).

Environmental Factors

Clearly not to be overlooked in psychiatric genetic counseling is the role of environmental influences on mood disorders. Environmental influences and experiences, including a variety of stresses, may play a critical part in the precipitation of a psychiatric illness, its degree of severity, and the potential for relapse, and may affect the response to treatment.

One very powerful indicator of environmental influences on the development of mood disorders is the lack of 100% concordance between monozygotic twins for affective illness, despite the fact that they possess identical genomes. One recent illustration that other factors must interact with genetic vulnerabilities is a case report involving identical twins with bipolar disorder. While both individuals had initial manic episodes within a year of each other, only one responded to lithium pharmacotherapy (Hoffman, 1987). Kraepelin (1921/1976), in his classic observations, described the role of stress in activating the illness in its earliest phases, and others have suggested more recently that the early intervention and resolution of environmental stressors may have a significant impact in preventing future episodes (Goodwin & Jamison, 1990). Reiss, Plonim, and Hetherington (1991) have argued that nonshared environmental effects—that is, the unique ways in which the environment (e.g., parents and peers) interacts with each sibling in a family—have been underappreciated and inadequately studied in the development of all forms of psychopathology.

A number of small studies have examined the effects on children of being raised by affectively ill parents. They found that maternal parenting deficits increase the risk to the children for impairments in affective regulation and social relations, as well as a range of diagnosable psychopathology (Davenport, Zahn-Waxler, Adland, & Mayfield, 1984; Gaensbauer, Harmon, Cytryn, & McKnew, 1984; Zahn-Waxler, McKnew, Cummings, Davenport, & Radke-Yarrow, 1984; Hammen et al., 1987). A recent study involving the Amish community supports the role of nongenetic maternal influences on the development of affective illness. Carter, Pauls, and Egeland (1992) found that the offspring of affectively ill mothers and of affectively ill fathers were at similar high risk when the parental psychiatric disorder was severe, for example, bipolar I disorder. However, when the parental affective illness was less severe, the offspring of affected mothers were at greater risk for illness than the offspring of affected fathers. As there is no difference in the rate of affective illness among all relatives of male and female probands in the Amish community, the researchers conclude that the family environment influences the expression of the underlying genetic vulnerability.

Environmental factors, such as seasonal variations in light and temperature, as well as disruption of the sleep-wake cycle, may also influence the expression of mood disorders (see review in Goodwin & Jamison, 1990). Affectively ill patients suffering with chronic medical illnesses, significant object loss, and other unsolvable life problems may not respond to otherwise adequate pharmacotherapy (Akiskal, 1982; Feinberg & Halbreich, 1985).

In summary, a great deal is still unknown about how environmental/developmental factors combine with genetic vulnerabilities to modify the expression of illness (Baron, 1991b). Nevertheless, the genetic counselor needs to appreciate what role stressors may have played in a given individual's illness, as well as communicate to a family how such stressors complicate risk prediction and adversely influence the course of the disorder.

GENETIC COUNSELING PROCESS

The purpose of psychiatric genetic counseling has been described as a means of providing scientifically valid information and advice to patients and their families within the context of a therapeutic relationship (Targum & Gershon, 1980). As Tsuang and Faraone (1990) note, genetic counseling helps people to be best prepared to cope with the adverse effect or possible recurrence of psychiatric illness. It alerts them to the possibility that an adolescent psychosis in the immediate family most likely is some form of mood disorder, and, therefore, is treatable.

While genetic counseling can be offered within the context of a short-term intervention such as psychoeducational work, or even a single consultation, genetic questions most often may be asked by patients and families at some point in the midst of ongoing therapy. In these situations, a well-prepared and knowledgeable therapist can incorporate genetic counseling into the therapeutic work (Targum, 1988; Gershon, 1990). If the therapist feels unable to address these issues within the treatment framework, referral to a psychiatrist experienced in genetic counseling is indicated.

Whether genetic questions are raised during ongoing treatment or as reason for consultation, the underpinning for the provision of effective counseling is a supportive therapeutic relationship that allows for an open dialogue among all involved (Targum & Gershon, 1980).

A systematic, stepwise approach to psychiatric genetic counseling derived from more general principles of medical genetic counseling (Feinberg, 1988; Targum, 1988; Targum & Gershon, 1980; Tsuang, 1978), serves as a template for performing this therapeutic work. We have found it helpful to use these steps as one might an outline of the mental status exam. Rigid adherence to this approach, just as to the mental status outline, can be awkward and lend a stilted character to the process, hindering the development of rapport. It may be more effective to integrate data collection, as well as the provision of information, into a more natural, flowing therapeutic process.

Steps in the Approach

1. *Assess the motive for seeking the genetic consultation or the raising of genetic issues during treatment.* The counseling professional has to understand who is doing the asking, why the person is asking, and why the questions are being raised at this point in therapy (Targum & Gershon, 1980). As a mental health professional, one is ideally suited to determine the stated purposes and concerns of the individuals who seek genetic counseling, as well as to appreciate the unconscious motivations that may be at play. Similarly, the raising of genetic concerns may serve a function within the family system that needs to be elucidated.

There are many possible motivations that should be considered. Is the patient concerned about the risk to any offspring? Is a patient seeking counseling because she is pregnant and is trying to determine whether or not to continue the pregnancy? Are patient and spouse considering adoption or artificial insemination to bypass the potential risk? However, the counselor also needs to weigh the possibility that the focus on hereditary risks is masking fears of parenthood or pregnancy.

An individual may request help because of his or her anxiety and fears about having, or being at risk for, a "genetic illness." Feeling helpless to control one's life against such an entity may, independently of the disorder itself, spawn depression or severe demoralization, and motivate one to seek clarification and guidance. In the same manner, a patient may seek counseling to integrate the experience of affective illness into a family historical context, to ease personal guilt, or to gain perspective on the impact of the illness on the person's life. Perhaps the patient hopes to minimize self-blame where he or she had previously viewed the symptoms as a sign of moral or other personal weakness. Alternatively, the motivation may be to externalize responsibility for one's actions ("It's the genetic illness") or to displace feelings of anger and guilt over life's difficulties onto other family members through rationalization, "*They* gave me this illness."

A prospective spouse may present when there is affective illness in the potential mate's family and desire counseling about the risk of illness to that person (Tsuang, 1978). A prospective or present spouse of a patient may be concerned about the genetic risk to children or the potential risk and consequences of the spouse's illness with regard to the person's ability to function as a parent. A spouse of an ill patient may be contemplating the possibility of getting a divorce. Alternatively, a young adult who is ambivalent about marriage for other, unconscious reasons may use this process to justify a life decision.

Families or individuals may come for genetic counseling when a near relative has become ill or when multiple family members have shown signs of illness. Their concern or curiosity may focus on themselves or others in the family. The parents and in-laws, caught up in the difficulties of their married children when one is ill, may be seeking to place blame for these problems on the other side of the family by demanding genetic counseling for the son-in-law or daughter-in-law.

Genetic questions may also come from a referring clinician who seeks assistance in establishing a diagnosis in an ambiguous case or direction toward a more efficacious medication. An adoption agency or parents considering adoption of a child from a psychiatrically ill mother may seek diagnostic and risk clarification (Targum, 1988).

The reasons why a person presents for counseling are sometimes evident, such as a life-cycle issues (e.g., marriage, childbirth) or a family crisis around an affective episode. As with any psychiatric consultation, though, it may take time to uncover the motivation that prompts a patient to seek help at a particular point in life. Understanding the underlying motivation is clearly an essential aspect of the counseling process.

Members of the Orthodox Jewish community may present with any of these motivations, with the exception of questions involving abortion, a practice forbidden by Jewish law, except in clear instances of life-threatening danger to the mother. Once married, unless one is extremely ill, the biblical priority to "be fruitful and multiply" will often overshadow concerns about any risk to future children. However, we have been involved in a number of cases where one or both partners in a couple have a malignant affective illness, and have entered into a discussion about the genetic aspects of the disorder in order to be able to bring this information to their rabbi (Feinberg, 1988). The rabbi then becomes, either directly or indirectly, a member of the consultation process and helps the couple to decide whether contraception is appropriate in their situation. This discussion often focuses on the present and long-term risk to the couple, or to the mother in dealing with the stresses of pregnancy, childbirth, and parenting, rather than the less clearly predictable risk to potential offspring.

As just discussed, questions about lineage are extremely important in this community, and genetic questions are frequently raised prior to marriage. In particular, we have found that not only will prospective spouses raise questions about the risk of illness in a potential mate and future children, but frequently the parents of the prospective spouse, their rabbi, or their matchmaker (the *shaddchen,*) will be the spokesperson for these concerns.

Alternatively, prior to pursuing marriage or undergoing the actual marriage ceremony, the individual with a history of a previous affective episode, or his or her family, will present in order to ascertain his or her potential for future illness. As the stigma around mental illness is especially great in this community, the hope may be to assess the feasibility of hiding this history from the potential spouse and family, if at all possible.

2. *Establish accurate diagnoses for the identified patient and family members.* Because the diagnosis of psychiatric disorders lacks the precision of many other medical illnesses, it is critical to use consistent clinical criteria (e.g., the revised third edition of the American Psychiatric Association's *Diagnostic and Statistical Manual of Mental Disorders*) to ascertain information about all involved individuals. The assessment consists of patient and family interviews, as well as a review of all available medical records, in order both to evaluate the cross-sectional clinical picture and to gather a longitudinal perspective on the course of the disorder (Tsuang, 1978).

In addition to a psychiatric history, one collects as much information as possible about first-and second-degree relatives, including their ages, sex, health status, medication use, cause of death, adoptions, and out-of-wedlock children (Tsuang, 1978). This information allows the construction of an accurate pedigree diagnosis.

The utilization of a semistructured clinical interview (e.g., the Schedule for Affective Disorders and Schizophrenia) has been suggested to ensure the rigorous collection of data during genetic research projects (Tsuang & Faraone, 1990; Endicott & Baron, 1994). However, this method of data collection does have limitations, especially when used by an inexperienced clinician (Endicott & Baron, 1994). Regardless of the type of interview employed, the interviewer, to ensure diagnostic accuracy, needs to follow up on any inconsistencies, or unclear issues that arise during the assessment. If uncertainty about the diagnosis of any individual still exists, this needs to be factored in and shared with the consultee, along with its implications for risk prediction (Tsuang & Faraone, 1990).

There are three other important considerations to keep in mind during the diagnostic assessment process, especially when reviewing past information. First, a given patient can present with different symptoms at different times because he or she has suffered from more than one psychiatric illness (e.g., an affective disorder and substance abuse) or has an illness with varying stages (e.g., bipolar disorder). A second consideration is the possibility that different clinicians may not have had the same database on which they formed their previous clinical impressions or, even having the same information, they may have reached different conclusions by organizing the clinical material in different manners (Spitzer, Endicott, & Robins, 1975). Finally, it has been demonstrated that gathering information through direct personal interviews (the family study method), in conjunction with a review of records and relative interviews, provides more accurate family diagnostic and rate-of-illness data than does family information collected through more indirect methods, that is, by asking relatives about the psychiatric history of other family member (the family history method of data collection) (Andreasen, Rice, Endicott, Reich, & Coryell, 1986). Therefore, it is useful to interview as many relatives as possible, especially closer first-degree relatives. In particular, interviewing multiple informants or a person who has lived with the individual being assessed will increase the likelihood of identifying the less dramatic affective disorders, such as dysthymia and cyclothymia.

In our work with the Orthodox Jewish community, we have encountered some interesting problems with this aspect of the process, though these issues are not necessarily unique to this population. As mentioned earlier, there is a great deal of fear, and thus denial, of psychiatric illness in this group (Feinberg, 1988). It is not uncommon to encounter these fears while trying to pull together pedigree information. The identified patients themselves may minimize valuable personal and family history. Other family members also may not be very forthcoming, if they are willing to talk at all. Taking the time to develop a trusting relationship, as well as seeking the support for this process from their rabbi, is sometimes, but not always, helpful. Sometimes the fear of exposure is too great to overcome.

The client's educational background and, in particular, knowledge of biology has been found by counselors to be a very common source of difficulty in problematic genetic consultations (Skinner, 1990). The less secularly educated members of the Orthodox Jewish community especially are not familiar with ordinary clinical terminology, symptoms, or concepts of affective illness. For example, families unfamiliar with bipolar disorder may have believed a hypomanic person's creative rationalizations for his or her episodic inappropriate and impulsive behavior. Therefore, it may not stand out in their minds as indicative of illness as you collect family history. Similarly, a man who episodically withdraws into the study of *musar* (ethics and moral perfection) may be seen as repenting or engaging in self-improvement. While this might well be the case, it can also be an indication of psychiatric illness, such as major depression or psychosis.

To collect accurate data, the counselor has to help the family members understand, in their own language, what types of information one is seeking. Listen for their unique "buzz" phrases, which may indicate signs or symptoms of clinical psychopathology. For example, hearing that someone at one time was "not learning," that is, unable to carry on the usual study of the Talmud in the presence of no known physical ailments, may indicate depression or psychosis. If a person suddenly starts sharing wild *chiddushim* (new ideas) in studying the Talmud, that raises the possibility of hypomania or psychosis. One is reminded here in some ways of the experiences of Dr. Janice Egeland and colleagues in ascertaining Amish pedigrees (Egeland, Hostetter, & Eshleman, 1983). They noted the Amish's descriptive terms for psychopathology, as well as their understanding at its origins.

Research from the Amish Study, as well as the "bipolar spectrum" concepts noted above, suggests that there is clear evidence for phenotypic heterogeneity—that a given pathogenic genotype may be expressed as one of several phenotypes. Therefore, to put together as accurate a pedigree as possible, it is important not to miss the identification of these spectrum disorders within a family. Knowledge about the variations of mood disorders also lends perspective and hope to families and individuals. Not all affective illness is an "out of control" psychotic mania or agitated, suicidal depression, but includes the milder, more subtle cyclothymic and hyperthymic temperaments, as well (Akiskal & Mallya, 1987).

Alcohol and substance abuse, frequently associated with mood disorders (Goodwin & Jamison, 1990), are found less commonly among Orthodox Jews (Feinberg & Feinberg, 1985). Thus the identification of an individual with alcohol or drug use in this community, as with the Amish, increases one's index of suspicion for affective illness.

3. *Estimate the risk in a given pedigree.* Once the diagnostic information about the pedigree has been collected and combined with empirical risk data, it is appropriate to address the questions that led to the request for counseling. As noted above, far from being an exact science, the word "estimate" best describes what a psychiatric genetic counselor can offer in terms of the prediction of occurrence in an unaffected individual and recurrence in one who has already manifested the illness (Tsuang & Faraone 1990). Follow-up studies on the effectiveness of genetic counseling indicate that great refinement of risk estimation may not in fact be crucial, as counselees often recall only the level of risk (high or low risk) of recurrence, rather than the actual numerical risk (Skinner, 1990).

It is prudent to consider the age of the individual at the time of assessment. That is, in a family at risk, a nonaffected individual at the age of 60 is at less risk than is a 15-year-old in the same family (Targum & Schulz, 1982). Also keep in mind that not all affective illness is necessarily hereditary, particularly where the pedigree is devoid of affective or affectively related illness (Targum & Gershon, 1980). Additionally, one needs to consider that there is a high frequency of assortative matings, and more specifically dual matings (mating of individuals who are both psychiatrically ill), which significantly increases the risk to offspring on a genetic basis, and probably on an environmental basis as well. (Merikangas, 1982; Targum & Schulz, 1982).

While a number of studies of varying methodological sophistication have suggested that being Jewish, and perhaps ultra-Orthodox, increases the incidence of affective illness (Gershon & Liebowitz, 1975; Cooklin, Ravindran, & Carney, 1983; Malzberg, 1973; Rahav, Goodman, Popper, & Lin, 1986), more recent epidemiologic work in Israel did not find this to be the case (Levav, 1991).

There is a tendency in some Hasidic families to marry relatives, such as first cousins. This raises the question of what effect consanguinity might have on the risk of affective illness in this group, or in any family. In general, consanguinity involving first cousins clearly increases the risk of disease produced by homozygosity for rare recessive genes, though the absolute risk of illness remains quite low (Vogel & Motulsky, 1986). For more common recessive conditions, it has been reported that the likelihood that the parents of a proband are consanguineous is no higher than that of parents of normal individuals (Pyeritz, 1991). An inbred group such as the Amish does not have a higher incidence of affective illness than the general population (Egeland & Hostetter, 1983).

4. *Assess the consultand's and family's concept of the burden of illness, capacity to comprehend the genetic information, and competence to make appropriate decisions.* The burden and risk of illness refer to the emotional, physical, and financial costs associated with the disorder for that particular person and family (Tsuang, 1978). Their importance as factors in the counseling process was evident in follow-up studies on the effectiveness of genetic counseling that found that the "burden" of illness is as influential as empirical risk information in the counselee's decision making (Skinner, 1990). Many variables affect the weight of the potential burden (Tsuang & Faraone, 1990). They include the degree of disruption and pain caused to date by mental illness; the potential consequences for the family of recurrence; the family members threshold for tolerating psychiatric illness; their coping style, personality, and defensive structure; and their religious convictions. In addition, the therapist should consider the size of the family, the couple's life expectations, the level of desire for children, and the partners perceptions of parenthood. Intelligence, educational background, family economic condition, direct medical costs, as well as indirect costs, incurred through the loss of employment or career,

and their support network, as well as the maturity and flexibility of the marriage, are additional variables that need to be examined.

A more severe psychotic form of affective illness or a refractory rapid cycling disorder carries with it a greater burden of illness (Targum & Gershon, 1980). What might appear to be the same types of burden can have quite a different impact on different individuals (Skinner, 1990). A spouse in one marriage may have a great deal of tolerance for, and even enjoy, a partner's hypomanic symptoms, whereas another spouse might find them intolerable (Targum & Gershon, 1980). This disparity in the perceptions of the burden of illness is also often evident in situations in which the patient denies the illness and its impact, while the family members who live and suffer with the person's disorder do not. This burden of illness is weighed against the very subjective benefits of taking a chance despite the illness, as by having a child or marrying an ill person.

The psychiatric counselor also needs to learn about a family's understanding of the disorder to appreciate to what extent they are able to process information offered them. Such variables as intelligence, level of insight, and defensive style (e.g., use of denial) are relevant here. Correspondingly, it is important to assess emotional state, judgment, and impulse control, including suicidality, before presenting any risk data. In essence, psychiatric genetic counselors have a responsibility to perform a mental status assessment on anyone they are counseling.

While it is incorrect to make generalizations about the entire Orthodox Jewish community, we have found that some burdens are especially great in Orthodox families. The infringement of critical Jewish laws and the family's public embarrassment during a psychotic manic episode, the endangerment of the family lineage, and the impact of psychiatric illness on the person's cognitive abilities all carry with them a large burden. Divorce in this community continues to take place far less frequently than in the general population and, when it does, it creates significant difficulty for all involved (Schindler, 1983). It, therefore, carries with it a heavy burden. On the benefit side of the burden/benefit ratio, both getting married and having children carry much weight.

5. *Communicate the genetic information.* Communication here entails a clear discussion of the nature and course of the illness, and

ideally should be employed as a part of an overall psychoeducational approach, as well as include a description of the genetic risk to all concerned. Early subtle signs of illness are described to help sensitize families to the onset of illness in a previously asymptomatic individual or as an indication of potential relapse (Fava & Kellner, 1991). Again, the information offered is based on what the counselor assesses the patient and family would like to learn, keeping in mind the elements described in the previous step. As Targum and Schulz (1982) emphasize, the dissemination of these genetic data requires delicate and cautious handling because of the potential effects on fragile individuals. It is not paternalistic to withhold information when the counselor feels it either is not relevant to the discussion or is beyond the comprehension or present emotional capacities of the individual. Risk data are probably best presented as a range of risk based on information such as offered in Table 8–1, as well as other gathered data as discussed (Tsuang & Faraone, 1990).

While a genetic counselor is often asked to describe the *exact* risk, the counselor's role is rather to help people become aware of the available information and to cope with the uncertainties that exist. Here, again, it is important to try to understand what specific concerns and fears underlie this question. This is further elaborated in the next step.

6. *Address individuals' feelings and concerns, especially in light of genetic information offered.* This step entails assisting individuals in their reconsideration of personal plans in view of the genetic risk information just communicated. In many ways, it can be the most difficult part of the process as the clinician brings together the knowledge gleaned from the other steps. Beyond his or her role as a presenter of information, the counselor is a supportive therapist encouraging the expression of fears and other feelings (Targum & Gershon, 1980). He or she may gently offer clarifications or interpretations to help an individual, a couple, or family members better appreciate what unconscious issues may be motivating their questions and underlie their anxiety. The counselor's role is to facilitate the working through of these feelings.

As discussed, a whole array of feelings may emerge, including anger, sadness, demoralization, and anxiety over being afflicted with, or being at risk for, a genetic illness. Addressing these feelings may remove a barrier or open up new avenues of exploration within an ongoing psychotherapy. Some people need help in mourning the loss of previous health, as one would grieve over other types of losses. Often, individuals are left to face an unsettling fear of the unknown as the counselor can only offer equivocal information on risk potential. Helping a family retain a reasonable level of concern while going on with the tasks of daily living is a desired goal (Papolos & Papolos, 1992). Alternatively, people may experience relief from self-blame, guilt, or exaggerated fears of future risks. Clients may feel hopeful after hearing that the risk of illness is many times less than the 50 to 100% risk frequently feared, as well as about the availability of potential treatments (Tsuang, 1978).

Orthodox Jewish families often respond with ambivalent, mixed feelings to the knowledge that affective disorder is a genetic illness with similarities to other medical illnesses. On the one hand, they are more comfortable with a disorder that is closely associated with the medical model of illness rather than with a "purely" psychological disorder. This is because they see the latter as based on psychodynamic thinking, a theoretical system that has challenged the legitimacy of their religious beliefs and practices (Feinberg & Feinberg, 1986). Yet, for reasons described earlier, Orthodox Jews greatly fear the stigmatization involved with an illness affecting the psyche that is *genetically* based. This fear of being stigmatized often has a basis in reality, and this clearly extends beyond the Orthodox Jewish community (e.g., see National Institute of Mental Health Conference Report, 1980). Part of the psychiatric counselor's function is to validate these concerns and help families to cope with this frustrating reality.

The client's reassessment of personal plans presents the counselor with a task that is somewhat similar to that of a psychotherapist who assesses which form of psychotherapy would be most appropriate for a given patient. Often, more highly functioning patients are given less specific advice and direction and are left to use their own coping skills, as in a more insight-oriented psychotherapy. The counselor may discuss the burden of illness, risk data, possible courses of action, and other relevant information. Many individuals are then quite capable of making their own life decisions. Patients with lesser ego strengths are provided with more concrete guidance in decision making, in keeping with a supportive mode of psychotherapy. This group may need very clear direction, such as being advised to postpone marriage or childbearing (Targum & Schulz, 1982). These recommendations may be offered when there is a dual mating and both spouses have significant psychotic illnesses, an individual has severe residual symptoms and dysfunction, a rapidly cycling bipolar illness is present, there is a frequent need for psychiatric hospitalization, or multiple suicide attempts have occurred. The counselor may be required to take clear-cut positions that involve life decisions when there is significant denial of illness and its likely negative consequences.

Among the possible motivations described, many involve decisions about family planning. In this context, it is important to note a study that involved directly questioning bipolar patients and their spouses. While only 5% of the bipolar patients expressed regrets over marrying or having children, about 53% of their spouses indicated that they would not have married had they known more about the illness beforehand (Targum, Dibble, Davenport, & Gershon, 1981). Furthermore, 47% of these spouses expressed regrets over having children.

A counselor may communicate to a couple concerned about adopting a child from a family with ill individuals that growing up in a supportive, nonstressful environment may attenuate the expression of psychiatric illness, but biological and genetic risk factors cannot be eliminated (Targum & Schulz, 1982). Through the description of empirical risk data and the concept of penetrance, the clinician can relate that the risk of developing illness may, in many cases, be quite low.

In the formulation of personal plans by an Orthodox Jewish family, a rabbi may be involved to help sort out the options from the perspective of Jewish law, as well as to offer more general counsel in formulating life choices (Feinberg, 1988). This has to be accepted and respected by the clinician, who may be asked to speak directly with the rabbi. Also, the rabbi may, if appropriate, join the actual counseling sessions.

One inference from our experience with this community, which applies to clinical work with all culturally distinct groups, is that the counselor needs to appreciate these cultural differences and their effects on the decision-making process. Although the conclusions reached may not be those desired by the clinician, he or she nevertheless must offer unbiased support. The following case example is illustrative.

A rabbi calls the counselor at the behest of a 37-year-old Orthodox Jewish mother of nine children, asking that she be evaluated as soon as possible. The counselor speaks briefly with the patient, who is obviously in the midst of an acute psychiatric episode, to set up the appointment. The patient is accompanied to the initial consultation by her mother. The history reveals symptoms consistent with an early manic episode with evidence of psychosis. On the mental status exam, the patient admits to auditory hallucinations and has grandiose ideas centered around her special relationship with God. The mother states that the patient had a psychotic episode at age 18, shortly before her marriage, which was responsive to antipsychotic pharmacotherapy. The medication was discontinued soon thereafter. At the age of 26, following the birth of a child, she had another episode, characterized by depressed mood, some confusion, and a decreased ability to handle responsibilities at home. The patient was again treated with antipsychotics prescribed by her internist and has continued on low-dose antipsychotics since that time. Her history over the years is also notable for some milder perturbations of mood that eventually resolved. Her husband is unaware of her psychiatric history, as the patient goes to her mother's house each day to take her medication, and has used a variety of excuses to explain previous difficulties. The patient is fearful that "he will divorce me if he finds out." In addition, any family history of psychiatric illness is quickly denied by both the mother and the daughter.

The presentation and previous history are consistent with a bipolar disorder. A description of the nature and course of bipolar illness and treatment alternatives is presented. The patient and her mother both vehemently veto any suggestion of hospitalization. As the patient's behavior is not out of control, there are no indications of suicidality, and she is willing to take medication, plans for outpatient treatment become the focus. A discussion about involving her husband in treatment reaches a compromise that, for the time being, the patient will only disclose to him her current situation and involve him in the ongoing treatment. The psychiatrist reluctantly agrees.

Subsequently, with appropriate pharmacotherapy, including lithium, as well as supportive psychotherapy with the family, the episode resolves and the patient returns to her baseline level of functioning. At this time, the patient, her husband, and her parents raise questions about genetic risk to the patient's children and future grandchildren, including her oldest daughter, who has recently been "matched" for marriage. A genetic assessment as per the above outline is given. Again, no psychiatric history is offered on either side of the family. Based on the available information, the potential burden of illness and estimated risk ranges are discussed. Despite the therapist's attempts, the patient continues to refuse to fully disclose her earlier psychiatric history to her husband. Treatment does help the patient and her spouse to accept the need to discuss openly the genetic risk issues with their oldest daughter. After weighing the pros and cons, their decision at this time is to not disclose any information to the daughter's suitor. They feel that if word of the illness were to spread, the entire family would be stigmatized, and the daughter's shiddach (potential marriage) would be endangered. The clinician empathizes with their concerns and leaves the door open for further discussion at a later time.

7. *Monitor the consultands over time to assess the outcome of counseling, as well as the course of illness and psychiatric status within the family.* The purpose of this step is to follow up on the client's understanding of the information discussed during the original consultation, and to be available for any additional questions. These may include questions related to changes in psychiatric status within the family that may affect risk estimates, the burden of illness, or life decisions (Tsuang & Faraone, 1990). While this is easily done within the context of ongoing treatment, it can also be done through follow-up consultations, telephone calls, or written communications. With some Orthodox consultands, we have found that follow-up discussions also allow for the uncovering of information consciously or unconsciously withheld earlier.

CONCLUSION

The process discussed, as part of a psychoeducational model, can be extremely important in helping to improve patients' and families' quality of life. Psychiatrists, perhaps more so than genetic counselors in other fields of medicine, possess the clinical skills necessary to provide these services effectively. Our experience with the Orthodox community emphasizes that the meaning of the term *genetic illness* to clients must be carefully assessed. Clinicians have the responsibility to understand the beliefs and culture of their patients in order to be most helpful to them.

As this book illustrates, this is an exciting, albeit somewhat confusing, time in psychiatric genetics. The explosion in psychiatric genetic knowledge will bring with it very serious ethical and clinical questions. Some of these are now being discussed in reference to such illnesses as Huntington's disease, where a greater fund of knowledge is available (Wexler, 1991). These ethical questions involve issues in genetic screening, and dilemmas about maintaining confidentiality, as well about defining one's responsibilities in the disclosure of information (Pardes et al., 1989; Shaw, 1990; Wexler, 1991). A full discussion of these issues is beyond the scope of this chapter. It is incumbent on the clinician to keep abreast of not just the most recent biological, genetic advances, but also of the ethical issues that will inevitably accompany them.

REFERENCES

Akiskal, H. S. (1982). Factors associated with incomplete recovery in primary depressive illness. *Journal of Clinical Psychiatry, 43,* 266–271.

Akiskal, H. S. (1983). The bipolar spectrum: New concepts in classification and diagnosis. In L. Grinspoon (Ed.), *Psychiatry update: The American Psychiatric Association annual review, Vol. II.* Washington, DC: American Psychiatric Association Press.

Akiskal, H. S., & Mallya, G. (1987). Criteria for the "soft" bipolar spectrum: Treatment implications. *Psychopharmacology Bulletin, 23,* 68–73.

Andreasen, N. C., Rice, J., Endicott, J., Coryell, W., Grove, W. M., & Reich, T. (1987). Familial rates of affective illness. *Archives of General Psychiatry, 44,* 461–469.

Andreasen, N. C., Rice, J., Endicott, J., Reich, T., & Coryell, W. (1986). The family history method to diagnosis: How useful is it? *Archives of General Psychiatry, 43,* 421–429.

Angst, J. (1961). A clinical analysis of the effects of Tofranil in depression. *Psychopharmacology, 2,* 381–407.

Baron, M., Risch, N., Hamburger, R., Mandel, B., Kushner, S., Newman, M., Drumer, D., & Belmaker, R. H. (1987). Genetic linkage between X-chromosome markers and bipolar affective illness. *Nature, 326,* 289–292.

Baron, M. (1991a). Genetics of manic-depressive illness: Current status and evolving concepts. In P. R. McHugh & V. A. McKusick (Eds.), *Genes, brain and behavior* (pp.153–163). New York: Raven.

Baron, M. (1991b). Genes, environment, and psychopathology. *Biological Psychiatry, 29,* 1055–1057.

Berrettini, W. H., Goldin, L. R., Gelernter, J., Gejman, P. V., Gershon, E. S., & Detera-Wadleigh, S. (1990). X-chromosome markers and manic-depressive illness: Rejection of linkage to Xq28 in nine bipolar pedigrees. *Archives of General Psychiatry, 47,* 366–373.

Biederman, J., Faraone, S. V., Keenan, K., & Tsuang, M. T. (1991). Evidence of familial association between attention deficit disorder and major affective disorders. *Archives of General Psychiatry, 48,* 633–642.

Campbell, J., Crowe, R. R., Goeken, N., Pfohl, B., Pauls, D., & Palmer, D. (1984). Affective disorders not linked to HLA in a large bipolar kindred. *Archives of General Psychiatry, 7,* 45–51.

Carter, A. S., Pauls, D. L., & Egeland, J. A. (1992). Differential risk for affective disorders among the Old Order Amish: An examination of the influence of maternal and paternal diagnostic status. Manuscript submitted for publication.

Cooklin, R. S., Ravindran, A., & Carney, M. W. P. (1983). The patterns of mental disorder in Jewish and non-Jewish admissions to a district general hospital psychiatric unit: Is manic-depressive illness a typically Jewish disorder? *Psychological Medicine, 13,* 209–212.

Davenport, Y. B., Zahn-Waxler, C., Adland, M. L., & Mayfield, A. (1984). Early child rearing practices in families with a manic-depressive parent. *American Journal of Psychiatry, 141,* 230–235.

Detera-Wadleigh, S. D., Berrettini, H., Goldin, L. R., Boorman, D., Anderson, C. M., & Gershon, E. S. (1987). Close linkage of c-Harvey-ras-1 and the insulin gene is ruled out in three North American pedigrees. *Nature, 325,* 806–808.

Egeland, J. A., & Hostetter, A. M. (1983). Amish Study I: Affective disorders among the Amish. *American Journal of Psychiatry, 140,* 56–61.

Egeland, J. A., Hostetter, A. M., & Eshleman, S. K., III. (1983). Amish Study, III: The impact of cultural factors on diagnosis of bipolar illness. *American Journal of Psychiatry, 140,* 67–71.

Egeland, J. A., Gerhard, D. S., Pauls, D. L., Sussex, J. N., Kidd, K. K., Allen, C. R., Hostetter, A. M., & Housman, D. E. (1987). Bipolar affective disorders linked to DNA markers on chromosome 11. *Nature, 325,* 783–787.

Endicott, J., & Baron, M. (1994). Diagnostic issues in pedigree assessment. In D. F. Papolos & H. Lachman, (Eds.), *Genetic studies in affective disorders.* New York: John Wiley.

Fava, G. A., & Kellner, R. (1991). Prodromal symptoms in affective disorders. *American Journal of Psychiatry, 148,* 823–830.

Feinberg, S. S. (1988, April). *A genetic disease: Bipolar disorder in the Orthodox Jewish community.* Presented at the first national conference of Orthodox psychotherapists, New York.

Feinberg, S. S. (1989, May). Treatment of the Orthodox Jewish patient: The Marpeh Clinic. In J. G. Bernstein (Chair.), *Treatment of the Orthodox Jewish Patient.* Workshop presentation at the 142nd annual meeting of the American Psychiatric Association, San Francisco, CA.

Feinberg, S. S., & Feinberg, K. G. (1985). An assessment of the mental health needs of the Orthodox Jewish population of metropolitan New York. *Journal of Jewish Communal Services, 62* (1), 29–39.

Feinberg, S. S., & Feinberg, K. G. (1986). The rabbi's view: On the mental health needs of Orthodox Jewish population. *Tradition, 22,* 82–94.

Feinberg, S. S., & Feinberg, K. G. (1987). Mental illness in Jerusalem. *American Journal of Psychiatry, 144,* 835–836.

Feinberg, S. S., & Halbreich, U. (1985). Management of treatment refractory depression: Evaluating the patient. *Drug Therapy, 15* (1), 121–134.

Feldman, D. M. (1974). *Marital relations, birth control and abortion in Jewish law.* New York: Schocken.

Gaensbauer, T. J., Harmon, R. J., Cytryn, L., & McKnew, D. H. (1984). Social and affective development in infants with a manic-depressive parent. *American Journal of Psychiatry, 141,* 223–229

Gershon, E. S. (1990). Genetics. In F. K. Goodwin & K. R. Jamison, (Eds.), *Manic-depressive illness* (pp. 373–401). New York: Oxford University Press.

Gershon, E. S., Hamovit, J., Guroff, J. J., Dibble, E., Leckman, J. F., Sceery, W., Targum, S. D., Nurnberger, J. I., Jr., Goldin, L. R., & Bunney, W. E. (1982). Family study of schizoaffective, bipolar, bipolar II, unipolar, and normal control probands. *Archives of General Psychiatry, 39,* 1157–1167.

Gershon, E. S., & Liebowitz, J. H. (1975). Sociocultural and demographic correlates of affective disorders in Jerusalem. *Journal of Psychiatric Research, 12,* 37–50.

Glassner, B., & Berg, B. (1984). Social locations and interpretations: How Jews define alcoholism. *Journal of Studies on Alcohol, 45,* 16–25.

Goodwin, F. K., & Jamison, K. R. (1990). *Manic-depressive illness.* New York: New York University Press.

Goshen-Gottstein, E. R. (1987). Mental health implications of living in an ultra-Orthodox Jewish subculture. *Israel Journal of Psychiatry and Related Sciences, 24,* 145–166.

Grunblatt, J. (1985, August). Psychiatry vis-à-vis the Torah tradition. In "Psychiatry and Orthodox ambivalence." Panel discussion presented at the annual convention of the Orthodox Jewish scientists, Spring Glen, NY.

Hammen, C., Gordon, G., Burge, D., Adrian, C., Jaenicke, C., & Hiroto, G. (1987). Maternal affective disorders, illness, and stress: Risk for children's psychopathology. *American Journal of Psychiatry, 144,* 736–741.

Hoffman, W. F. (1987). Identical twins' nonresponses to lithium. *American Journal of Psychiatry, 144,* 1240–1241.

Hudson, J. I., & Pope, H. G., Jr. (1990). Affective spectrum disorder: Does antidepressant response identify a family of disorders with a common pathophysiology? *American Journal of Psychiatry, 147,* 552–564.

Kelsoe, J. R., Ginns, E. E., Egeland, J. A., Gerhard, D. S., Goldstein, A. M., Bale, S. J., Pauls, D. L., Long, R. T., Kidd, K. K., Conte, G., Housman, D. E., & Paul, S. (1989). Re-evaluation of the linkage relationship between chromosome 11p loci and the gene for bipolar affective disorder in the Old Order Amish. *Nature, 342,* 238–243.

Kraepelin, E. P. (1921). *Manic-depressive insanity and paranoia.* (R. M. Barclay, Trans., & G. M. Robertson, Ed.). Edinburgh, Scotland: Livingstone. (Reprinted New York: Arno Press, 1976.)

Kutcher, S., & Marton, P. (1991). Affective disorders in first-degree relatives of adolescent onset bipolars, unipolars, and normal controls. *Journal of the American Academy of Child and Adolescent Psychiatry, 30,* 75–78.

Leckman, J. F., Gershon, E. S., McGinniss, M. H., Targum, S. D., & Dibble, E. D. (1979). New data do not suggest linkage between the Xg blood group and bipolar illness. *Archives of General Psychiatry, 36,* 1435–1441.

Levav, I. (1991). Current prevalence of psychiatric disorders. In A. E. Skodol (Chair.), *Mental disorders in Israel: An epidemiologic study.* Symposium presented at the 144th annual meeting of the American Psychiatric Association, San Francisco, CA.

Levitz, I. N. (1979). Orthodoxy and mental health: Suggested parameters for empirical study. *Journal of Psychology and Judaism, 4,* 87–99.

Liebman, C. S. (1983). Orthodox Judaism today. In R. P. Bulka (Ed.), *Dimensions of Orthodox Judaism* (pp. 106–120). New York: KTAV.

Malzberg, B. (1973). Mental disease among Jews in New York State. *Acta Psychiatrica Scandinavica, 49,* 479.

Mendlewicz, J., Fieve, R., & Stallone, F. (1973). Relationship between the effectiveness of lithium therapy and family history. *American Journal of Psychiatry, 130,* 1011–1013.

Merikangas, K. R. (1982). Assortative mating for psychiatric disorders and psychological traits. *Archives of General Psychiatry, 39,* 1173–1180.

Morton, N. E., & Maclean, C. J. (1974). Analysis of family resemblance: III. Complex segregation analysis of quantitative traits. *American Journal of Human Genetics, 26,* 489–503.

National Institute of Mental Health Conference Report. (1980). Stigma: Its impact on the mentally ill. *Hospital and Community Psychiatry, 31,* 342–346.

Nurnberger, J. I., Jr., (1987). Pharmacogenetics of psychoactive drugs. *Journal of Psychiatric Research, 21,* 499–505.

Papolos, D., & Papolos, J. (1992). *Overcoming depression.* New York: Harper/Collins.

Pardes, H., Kaufmann, C. A., Pincus, H. A., & West, A. (1989). Genetics and psychiatry. Past discoveries, current dilemmas, and future directions. *American Journal of Psychiatry, 146,* 435–443.

Pare, C. M. B., & Mack, J. W. (1971). Differentiation of two genetically specific types of depression by the response to antidepressant drugs. *Journal of Medical Genetics, 8,* 306–309.

Price, J. (1968). The genetics of depressive behavior. In A. Coppen & A. Walk (Eds.), *Recent developments in affective disorders* (pp. 37–54). *British Journal of Psychiatry* (Special Publisher 2).

Pyeritz, R. E. (1991). Formal genetics in humans: Mendelian and non-Mendelian inheritance. In P. R. McHugh & V. A. McKusick (Eds.), *Genes, brain, and behavior* (pp. 47–73). New York: Raven.

Rahav, M., Goodman, A. B., Popper, M., & Lin, S. P. (1986). Distribution of treated mental illness in the neighborhoods of Jerusalem. *American Journal of Psychiatry, 143,* 1249–1254.

Reiss, D., Plonim, R., & Hetherington, E. M. (1991). Genetics and psychiatry: An unheralded window on the environment. *American Journal of Psychiatry, 148,* 283–291.

Rice, J., Reich, T., Andeasen, N. C., Endicott, J., Van Eerdewegh, M., Fishman, R., Hirschfeld, R. M., & Klerman, G. L. (1987). The familial transmission of bipolar illness. *Archives of General Psychiatry, 44,* 441–447.

Schindler, R. (1983). Counseling Hasidic couples: The cultural dimension. *Journal of Psychology and Judaism, 8* (1), 52–61.

Schlesser, M. A., & Altshuler, K. Z. (1983). The genetics of affective disorder: Data, theory and clinical applications. *Hospital and Community Psychiatry, 34,* 415–422.

Shaw, M. W. (1990). Legal considerations in the delivery of genetic care. In A. E. H. Emery & D. L. Rimoin (Eds.), *Principles and practice of medical genetics* (pp. 2017–2023). New York: Churchill Livingstone.

Skinner, R. (1990). Genetic counseling. In A. E. H. Emery & D. L. Rimoin, (Eds.), *Principles and practice of medical genetics* (pp. 1923–1933). New York: Churchill Livingstone.

Slater, E., & Tsuang, M. T. (1968). Abnormality on maternal and paternal sides: Observations on schizophrenia and manic-depression. *Journal of Medical Genetics, 5,* 197–199.

Spitzer, R. L., Endicott, J., & Robins, E. L. (1975). Reliability of clinical criteria for psychiatric diagnosis. *American Journal of Psychiatry, 132,* 1187–1192.

Targum, S. D. (1988). Genetic issues in treatment. In J. F. Clarkin, G. L. Haas, & I. D. Glick (Eds.), *Affective disorder and the family: Assessment and treatment* (pp. 196–212). New York: Guilford.

Targum, S. D., Dibble, E. D., Davenport, Y. B., & Gershon, E. S. (1981). Family attitudes questionnaire: Patients and spouse view bipolar illness. *Archives of General Psychiatry, 38,* 562–568.

Targum, S. D., & Gershon, E. S. (1980). Genetic counseling for affective illness. In R. Belmaker & H. van Praag (Eds.), *Mania: An evolving concept* (pp. 119–126). Holliswood, NY: Spectrum.

Targum, S. D., & Schulz, S. C. (1982). Clinical applications of psychiatric genetics. *American Journal of Orthopsychiatry, 52,* 45–57.

Tsuang, M. T. (1978). Genetic counseling for psychiatric patients and their families. *American Journal of Psychiatry, 135,* 1465–1475.

Tsuang, M. T., & Faraone, S. V. (1990). *The genetics of mood disorders.* Baltimore, MD: Johns Hopkins University Press.

Turner, W. J., & King, S. (1983). BPD2: An autosomal dominant form of bipolar affective disorder. *Biological Psychiatry, 18,* 63–87.

Vogel, F., & Motulsky, A. G. (1986). *Human genetics.* Berlin: Springer-Verlag.

Weissman, M. M., Leaf, P. J., Tischler, G. L., Blazer, D. B., Karno, M., Livingston Bruce, M., & Florio, L. P. (1988). Affective disorders in five United States communities. *Psychological Medicine, 18,* 141–153.

Wexler, N. (1991). Ethical issues arising from the study of Huntington's disease. In C. N. Pato (Chair.), *Ethical issues of genetic research in psychiatry.* Symposium presented at the 144th annual meeting of the American Psychiatric Association, San Francisco, CA.

Wikler, M. (1979). The recent rise of professional Orthodox Jewish social services. *Journal of Jewish Communal Services, 55,* 279–284.

Zahn-Waxler, C., McKnew, D., Cummings, E. M., Davenport, Y. B., & Radke-Yarrow, M. (1984). Problem behaviors in peer interaction of young children with a manic-depressive parent. *American Journal of Psychiatry, 141,* 236–240.

PART III
Animal Models and In Vitro Systems: Future Directions

9

Animal Models in the Study of Genetic Factors in Human Psychopathology

FRITZ A. HENN AND
EMMELINE EDWARDS

DEVELOPMENT OF ANIMAL MODELS BASED ON BEHAVIORAL FEATURES OF HUMAN DISEASE

The development of animal models that embody aspects of human psychopathology affords the opportunity to study both the neuroanatomical structure that underlies specific behaviors and the effects of pharmacological agents that act on these behaviors. The establishment of an animal model for a condition that has its principal manifestations within the domain of subjective feelings, thoughts, or sensory impressions poses considerable obstacles. Yet, if we are ever to develop a truly functional neuroanatomy of psychiatric illness, the development of such models is a vital and necessary task.

The most plausible and efficient means to develop an animal model for a specific and well-defined behavioral condition is to attempt to reproduce specific behaviors that constitute the central features of the human condition. This suggests that we need not reproduce the forme fruste of mania, depression, or schizophrenia in animals, but rather concentrate on the establishment of a model and the understanding of central mechanisms that regulate or influence core behaviors in these

---

Supported by National Institute of Mental Health Physician Scientist Research Development Award 1K20MH00873-01A2 and by a NARSAD Young Investigator Award.

conditions, such as hedonic tone, libido, appetite, activity, sleep, memory, and social behavior. Such a model would ultimately encompass the genetic substrate that gives rise to these behaviors, take into account the complexity and uniquely human aspects of psychopathology, and yet also recognize that certain common behavioral repertoires that persist throughout evolution can be usefully studied in an animal species.

AN ANIMAL MODEL OF DEPRESSION: "LEARNED HELPLESSNESS"

We have chosen to focus on the "learned helplessness" model, initially developed by Overmeier and Seligman (1967). This model, in our hands, has been developed to mimic depressive illness. On theoretical grounds, the model rests firmly on the cognitive theory of depression developed by Beck. In addition to our work (Henn, Johnson, Edwards, & Anderson, 1985), Weiss and colleagues (1981) have found that the helpless state is one in which a variety of neurovegetative symptoms are expressed. The central feature of the model is the learned response of an animal to an uncontrollable stressor. The lack of an attempt to overcome such stressors (even those that can be avoided) after sufficient prior exposure to unavoidable and uncontrollable stressors is the defining behavioral characteristic of the model. We have utilized this model in order to study the central mechanism or mechanisms that underlie mood regulation.

Within this paradigm, a rat is exposed to uncontrollable foot shock for half of a 40-minute training period. On the following day, the animal is tested by exposure to 15 foot shock trials that can be terminated if the animal presses a bar. Animals that do not learn this task within 10 trials are considered learned helpless (LH), animals that learn the task within 5 trials are *not* considered helpless and are termed non-learned helpless (NLH). In initial studies, a triadic design was utilized. An "executive" control animal received the same amount of footshock as the experimental animal, except that the executive could terminate the shock via an active bar press and escape, whereas the barpress in the experimental animal's cage was inactive—making the shock inescapable. The difference between the executive and experimental animals did not reside in exposure or lack of exposure to shock, but rather in the ability of the animals to control the shock. The executive controls did not become helpless, as originally demonstrated by Weiss and colleagues (1982).

Helpless animals appear to share a number of behavioral features in common with humans who experience clinical depression. Because a practical test of an animal model for a condition whose etiology is unknown involves both phenomenological similarity to the condition being modeled and similar treatment responses, we first examined standard vegetative behaviors in the helpless animals, including sleep, appetite, motor activity, and libido. We found a disturbance in the sleep-wake cycle in helpless animals, an observation that was later confirmed by other investigators (Adrien, Dugovic, & Martin, 1991). In addition, we found a greater degree of weight loss and a slower recovery of weight in helpless animals as compared with controls. Libido was tested by exposing males to estrous females and counting offspring. The helpless animals produced only a tenth the number of offspring as the control animals. In tests of motor activity, the animals appeared agitated and exhibited less purposeful, more aimless movements. Thus these animals were observed to share a variety of signs and symptoms commonly seen in patients who suffer clinical depressions and severe anxiety states.

EFFECT OF PSYCHOTROPIC DRUG TREATMENTS

We also examined the effects of a variety of treatment approaches on helpless behavior. When treated chronically with standard antidepressant drugs (Table 9–1), the learned response to uncontrollable shock in LH animals can be reversed. A single dose of a standard pharmacological treatment for depression, tricyclic antidepressant drugs, however, has no effect on the behavior. Rather, the animals respond to the medication over four to five days, analogous to the 7 to 14 day period observed in the clinical response of human depression with these same agents. The classical tricyclic antidepressants and monoamine oxidase inhibitors (MAOIs) all appear to reverse helpless behavior. The blood levels required to achieve this effect are within the established therapeutic range for clinical populations that respond to an antidepressant

TABLE 9–1
Effectiveness of Various Treatments in Reversing Helpless Behavior

Effective	Ineffective
Tricyclic antidepressants	Antipsychotics
Monoamine oxidase inhibitors	Sedatives
5HT$_{1B}$ reuptake inhibitors	Barbiturates
Electroconvulsive therapy	Benzodiazepines
Atypical antidepressants	Anesthetics

trial. Atypical antidepressants such as trazodone, mianserin and fluoxetine are also effective in reversing helpless behavior. Classes of compounds that are not effective include benzodiazepines, sedatives, and antipsychotics, including phenothiazines and butyrophenones. Thus learned helpless behavior in rats appears to meet the criteria for a practical model of mood disorders.

THE NEUROCHEMICAL ANATOMY OF MELANCHOLIA

Having first established the distinguishing characteristics of the model, we attempted to define the neurochemical anatomy of the circuits involved in the establishment of helpless behavior. Initially, we felt that by defining the receptor changes that occur after the induction of helplessness, we might be able to outline the neurochemical circuit that regulates this behavior. To initiate this aspect of the study, we measured amine and amino-acid receptors across 17 brain regions. These studies revealed that there did exist very specific changes in well-defined neuroanatomical regions that correlate with the induction and maintenance of learned helpless behavior.

With regard to dopamine, there do not appear to be significant changes in receptor function within any brain region that we studied, whereas the up-regulation of β-adrenergic receptors in the hippocampus and their corresponding down-regulation in the hypothalamus (Martin, Edwards, Johnson, & Henn, 1990) could be consistently reproduced experimentally. Additionally, decreased activity of the α_2 1-1 adreno-receptors in the locus coeruleus has been reported in the

LH model, which can be reversed by agonist microinfusion (Simson, Weiss, Hoffman, & Ambrose, 1986). Since it has been found that, in some groups of individuals, low cerebrospinal levels of serotonin are associated with suicidal (Asberg, Traskman, & Thoren, 1976) and impulsive behaviors (Linnoila et al., 1983), we have begun to examine the contribution of the serotonergic (5-HTergic) system to learned helplessness. As noted previously, selective serotonin (5-HT) reuptake inhibitors have been found to be effective clinical antidepressants and also to reverse helpless behavior. The 5-HT reuptake system that involves the 5-HT_{1b} receptor has been examined in both LH and NLH animals. The LH animals were found to have altered 5-HT_{1b} receptors in the hippocampus and hypothalamus, with up-regulation seen in the hippocampus and down-regulation observed in the hypothalamus (Edwards, Harkins, Wright, & Henn, 1991). These changes in 5-HT_{1b} receptor density parallel the β-adrenergic receptor findings, and point to the role of both neurotransmitter systems in the regulation of the limbic circuit-hypothalamic–pituitary axis (HPA), as well as to their influence on LH behavior.

One final receptor difference of significance has been documented in LH animals. Rather unexpectedly, we observed changes in cortical and subcortical μ-opiate receptor density in the LH strain. The LH animals appear to have higher levels of μ-opiate receptors in the cortical, hippocampal, and septal regions selectively (Edwards, Muneyyirci, van Houten, Michel, & Henn, 1991).

These results have allowed us to formulate a tentative neurochemical anatomy of helplessness that has some features in common with the hypothetical circuit for emotion originally proposed by the neuroanatomist James Papez (1937). The limbic forebrain provides a key integrating system for selectively modulating emotion and responses to physical sensations. Its unique location within the forward part of the brain enables it to correlate and integrate every form of internal and external perception. It is the interconnections between various limbic and hypothalamic centers that led Papez to propose this particular anatomical circuit as a neuronal substrate of emotion. To support the claim that these structures formed a circuit that permitted emotion to arise through neuronal activity in the limbic system, he noted the association between the essential lesions of rabies, the Negri bodies, which are most abundant in the hippocampus, and the intense behavioral and emotional symptoms that occur in the early stages of the disease. Insomnia, irritability, and restlessness typically usher in the stage of excitement and profound mood lability, as well as excruciating sensitivity to all forms of stimuli, such as light and sound.

Our experimental findings with an animal model of depression indicate that the hippocampus is also central to the processing of neural input, which leads to helpless behavior. Information is relayed via the fornix, a system that represents the major pathway for the interconnection of the septohippocampal complex with the hypothalamus and midbrain. Through this bundle of fibers, neuronal information from hippocampal regions gains access to the septum and higher cortical regions, as well as the stress-responsive HPA. Behavioral functions regulated by hypothalamic centers are clearly altered in LH animals. In addition, the hippocampus is the richest central site for glucocorticoid receptors. These receptors provide a target for feedback into the Central Nervous System (CNS) by the HPA. Taken together, these observations suggest that all the components for interaction between the HPA and the limbic circuit mediating emotional response to external stimuli are present. Indeed, there is some experimental support for the possibility that such a circuit influences LH behavior.

Early lesion studies have implicated the activity of the fornix in helpless behavior (Leshner & Segal, 1979). Transection of the fornix blocks the development of learned helplessness in rats. The inhibitory transmitter aminobutyric acid (GABA) appears to be the principal neurotransmitter that is active in this part of the limbic–hypothalamic circuit. Furthermore, we have found that LH animals are sensitive to manipulations of the HPA. Following adrenalectomy, a far higher percentage of animals than is ordinarily observed become spontaneously helpless, an effect that can be reversed by corticosterone replacement (Edwards, Harkins, Wright, & Henn 1990). This demonstrates that the central circuit that regulates the expression of helpless behavior is responsive to changes in the HPA and supports the existence of a sensitive fast 1–1 feedback loop between adrenal corticosterone release, limbic activity, and hypothalamic release of corticotropin releasing factor (CRF). A rate-sensitive fast-feedback inhibition of stress-induced CRF secretion by glucocorticodis is well documented in rats

(Sapolsky & Plotsky, 1990; Young, Murphy-Weinberg, Haskett, Watson, & Akil, 1991). Such a phenomenon, however, only recently has been demonstrated in human subjects and notably was found to be absent in patients with major depression (Young et al., 1991). These data of altered fast-feedback regulation in depression lend further support to the hypothesis that alterations of glucocorticoid receptors at the level of the hippocampus may be involved in the HPA dysregulation in depression.

Many depressed patients have cortisol rhythms that do not manifest the expected circadian pattern, and also reach higher average levels than those seen in healthy controls (Sachar et al., 1973). This clinical finding was exploited with the development of the dexamethasone suppression test in which a dose of dexamethasone was administered in the evening and cortisol levels measured the following morning and afternoon. Control subjects manifest profound depression of endogenous cortisol, while several other groups, including patients with major depression, anorexia, and Alzheimer's disease, fail fully to suppress the production of cortisol. We examined the ability of helpless animals to suppress corticosterone production following dexamethasone in comparison with control animals (Greenberg, Edwards, & Henn, 1989). The helpless animals, as shown in Figure 9–1, do not suppress corticosterone release in response to stressors to the same degree as control animals, which reveals yet another parallel between the animal model and the clinical disorder. Through other experiments in which animals were adrenalectomized, we have shown that a lack of corticosterone results in an enhancement of helpless behavior, and, conversely, that the induction of LH behavior in an intact animal leads to a loss of feedback regulation of corticosterone production or release. To further examine the responsiveness of the HPA in LH animals, we exposed both control animals and helpless animals to a strong stressor, immobilization stress. We unexpectedly found that the control animals were able to elevate their corticosterone levels to a considerably higher degree in response to stress than the helpless animals. This suggests that the up-regulation of steroid production in response to stress is also disturbed in LH animals. The fact that both up- and down-regulation are impaired in LH animals implies that the HPA, a natural homeostatic system that buffers stress, functions poorly in helpless animals.

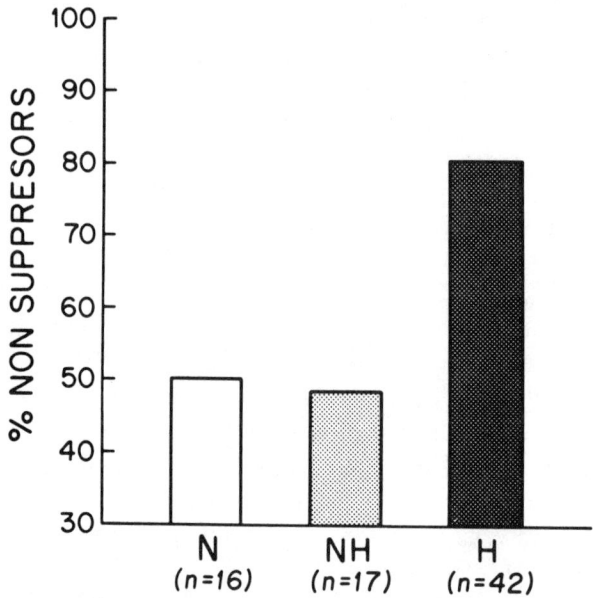

Figure 9–1. Animals were pretreated with 100 μg/g of dexamethasone, blood samples were taken 24 hrs later and plasma corticosterone measured. We defined suppression as a corticosterone level below 150 mg/ml following dexamethasone.

Therefore, the lack of a functional HPA can lead to helplessness, and conversely, helplessness leads to an ineffective HPA response to stress—a reciprocal relationship pointing to the tight interplay between the HPA and the central mechanisms that regulate mood.

The neurochemical systems involved in LH behavior appear to be specific and to involve an up-regulation of β-adrenergic receptors only within the hippocampus, while 5-HT re-uptake systems are altered in the hippocampus, septum, and anterior neocortex. In receptor studies of suicide victims, β-adrenergic receptor changes have been found in anterior neocortex, as well as in the hippocampus. These findings are consistent with the evolution of the human neocortex, which assumes some of the associative functions carried out in the hippocampus of lower vertebrates. In general, studies of completed suicides, which are closely related to depressive illness, also report changes in the β-adrenergic receptor (Mann, Stanley, McBride, & McEwen, 1986), the 5-HT uptake receptor (Gross-Isseroff, Salma, Israeli, & Biegon, 1989), and the μ-opiate receptor (Gross-Isseroff, Dillon, Israeli, & Biegon, 1990).

The next question is, which of these systems provides the substrate for antidepressant activity? Is there a general pattern of response to antidepressant treatments or do different treatments act on different systems? Since many antidepressants are thought to act via the down-regulation of the β-adrenergic receptor, we examined the temporal relationship between the reversal of learned helpless behavior and β-adrenergic receptor changes in LH animals. We found that imipramine does indeed result in down-regulation of the hippocampal β-receptors within the same five-day period necessary to reverse the learning deficit observed in helpless animals. In an effort to determine whether a close correlation existed between helpless behavior and β-adrenergic receptor up-regulation, we examined a large group of helpless rats over time. The propensity to develop helpless behavior is time limited. If the animals are not exposed to inescapable stressors following their initial training exposure, LH rats revert to normal behavior after three to four weeks. We next studied a proportion of helpless animals at increasingly longer intervals, and checked their behavioral responses and then the density of hippocampal β-adrenergic receptors. In all experiments performed, the results revealed a remarkably tight correlation ($r > 0.9$) between the level of β-adrenergic receptors and the expression of helpless behavior.

Having established this close correlation between up-regulated β-adrenergic receptors and helpless behavior, we sought to evaluate other antidepressant treatments that are thought to act exclusively through the 5-HTergic system, with little, if any, effect on β-adrenergic receptors. Mianserin, an antidepressant agent reported to act primarily on 5-HT receptors as well as via α-2 adrenergic receptors, and fluoxetine, a specific 5-HT re-uptake receptor blocker, were chosen. Mianserin is an effective antidepressant that is widely used in Europe, and when given chronically to rats, has been reported not to cause down-regulation of β-adrenergic receptors (Mishra, Janowsky, & Sulser, 1980). Yet our studies found that this drug was also effective in reversing helplessness and caused down-regulation of β-adrenergic receptors as effectively as imipramine when administered to helpless animals.

Animal Models and In Vitro Systems

However, mianserin did not down-regulate β-adrenergic receptors in untrained, naive animals. These findings suggest that the pathological up-regulation of hippocampal β-adrenergic receptors in LH animals is sensitive to control through some action of mianserin, a phenomenon not observed when the drug is administered to normal animals. We also found selective 5-HT reuptake inhibitors such as fluvoxamine (Figure 9–2) to be effective in reversing helpless behavior. This class of drugs appears to be specific for 5-HT reuptake and purportedly do not affect the noradrenergic system. Again we found that β-adrenergic receptors were down-regulated in animals that reverted to normal behavior following fluvoxamine treatment. This strongly suggests that in the pathological condition of helplessness, the hippocampal neurons that contain β-adrenergic receptors must be regulated not only by

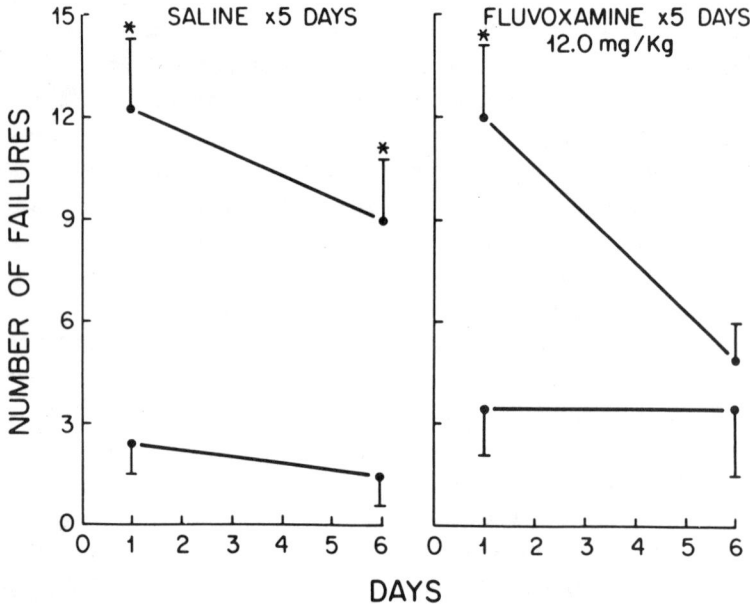

Figure 9–2. Six animals in both groups were trained and tested to meet helpless criteria. One group was given IP saline and the other IP fluvoxamine for 5 days and retested for helplessness. The fluvoxamine group showed a significant reversal of behavior.

presynaptic levels of norepinephrine, but also by 5-HT effects on β-adrenergic receptor activity. Such a possibility was originally proposed by Janowsky, Okada, Manier, Applegate, and Sulser, (1982) and supported by the work of Stockmeier, Martino, and Kellar (1985), who found that 5-HT innervation was necessary for β-receptor regulation, but then called this into question because of problems with endogenous ligand present during the binding studies. It appears that there may exist some discrete differences between the mechanisms that control the functional levels of β-adrenergic receptors in normal and pathological hippocampal tissue slices. Our data further suggest that 5-HT may play a major role in the control of β-adrenergic receptors in the helpless state, and that a common correlate of all treatments that reverse helpless behavior is the reduction of β-adrenergic receptors in hippocampal tissue. By analogy, the down-regulation of β-adrenergic receptors may be a common correlate of all clinically effective antidepressant treatments.

USE OF ANIMAL MODELS TO STUDY GENETIC VULNERABILITY

The generation of hypotheses about the anatomy of melancholia and the general features of antidepressant response in humans shows one aspect of the utility of animal models. However, we suspect that human psychopathology is the result of a complex interplay between environmental factors and genetic susceptibility. Can animal models be used to help tease apart these factors? In the learned helpless model, we have a prime example of the way in which a particular environmental stress can lead to altered, pathological behavior in the animal. We have reviewed the evidence that shows that the crucial feature in the induction of helplessness is the perception of lack of control, a psychological stressor. This psychological stressor appears to interact with a given animal's genetic vulnerability. As many as 80% of normal rats do not develop helpless behavior following a 40 1-1 minute training period, and animals obtained from different suppliers become helpless at varying rates. These strain-to-strain differences led us to postulate that different strains of animals have variable susceptibilities to uncontrolled stress and that this may reflect a different underlying genetic makeup. It should, therefore, be possible to breed selected lines with greater susceptibility to an uncontrollable stressor.

We began to test this hypothesis by inbreeding animals that demonstrated a greater susceptibility to developing helplessness. Inbreeding biologically related LH animals will tend to move all genes toward a homozygous state, those involved in the susceptibility for the development of helplessness and all others in the genome of the sibs. Whereas selective lines that use unrelated animals that express the trait of interest (the susceptibility to becoming helpless after exposure to uncontrollable stress) result in a concentration of phenotypically relevant genes toward a homozygous state, all other genes maintain genetic variability. After reviewing work on quantitative animal behavioral genetics we chose to use a selective breeding strategy rather than inbreeding. This strategy has been particularly successful in studies of ethanol-sensitive and 1-1insensitive mice (Sorensen, Palmer, Dunwiddie, & Hoffer, 1980). By breeding unrelated animals that express the LH phenotype, a line should result in which the ensemble of genes that are associated with the behavior is concentrated. Conversely, breeding unrelated animals that do not exhibit the behavior should result in a line that is uniformly resistant to that behavior. The difference between these lines should be entirely attributable to the genes that regulate the behavior in question, while the transmission of all other genes should remain random. This model provides the ideal substrate for studying the genetic factors involved in the behavior of interest.

We have established animal lines for the susceptibility to learned helplessness and now have lines that have been bred for over 20 generations. This endeavor has resulted in a susceptible line that spontaneously expresses helpless behavior without a training session. How might this development relate to the problem of genetic linkage in depression? One problem with classical linkage analysis is the need to specify a model of gene transmission. Usually, one dominant gene—and almost always three or fewer genes—is assumed to account for the human disease. While this is certainly reasonable for many human genetic diseases, it may not be the case for many behavioral conditions. To date, family and linkage studies of depressive illness have not been able to determine unequivocally whether the condition can be represented by a single gene model or a polygenic model.

One way of conceptualizing anxiety and depressive illnesses involves the assumption that there are partially related multigene disorders. Here we have some number of genes (hypothetically eight in the figure) that combine in different assortments to yield a variety of phenotypic outcomes. Each gene makes a protein, which, in turn, acts with other proteins to carry out some specific physiological function. These physiological functions interact to result in specific behaviors, and groups of these behaviors interact to lead to psychiatric syndromes. While such a construct is speculative, it might be testable using the approaches developed by behavioral genetics. If our animal model of depression does involve some of the behavioral features that characterize human depression, then the genes that express the specific proteins that regulate LH behavior should be preferentially expressed in the strain that is susceptible to uncontrollable stressors, and should be distinguishable on this basis from the NLH strain.

Since we have been able to produce a strain of animals that is spontaneously helpless, it may be that some genetic elements common to human depressive or anxiety disorders have been differentially expressed in this strain as compared with the resistant strain. As an initial test of this hypothesis, we looked at the receptors that appear to be altered in helpless animals as compared with controls. As expected, the spontaneously helpless LH strain exhibited receptor changes previously seen with induced helpless behavior. The problem is that these changes could be secondary to a fundamental alteration in gene expression involving some unknown element. This is, in fact, likely to be the case for small changes in the range of 25% to 50% of baseline. All the changes noted in the noradrenergic and 5-HT systems are within this range, which indicates that these homeostatic CNS modulating systems are probably responding to a more fundamental alteration.

The most robust receptor change found in studies of LH animals was the change in the expression of μ-opiate receptors. These receptors appear to be approximately two- to threefold greater in selected regions of the spontaneously helpless animals as compared with the resistant line or controls. This is a significant alteration and suggests a possible trait marker.

While this finding requires replication, it is nevertheless of interest that the changes reported by Gross-Isseroff et al. (1990) for the μ-

receptor density in the brains of young suicide victims were more than ninefold higher than the levels seen in control brains. This is indeed a remarkable difference for a finding in biological psychiatry, and suggests that μ-receptor levels should be examined as a function of the depressed state and as a trait marker in families with clear histories of endogenous depression. It also offers a potential avenue for developing therapeutic agents for depression.

To take full advantage of the strain differences we have observed, a systematic examination of gene expression in the two strains should be carried out, and, in addition, subtraction libraries should be constructed to pinpoint the major differences in genetic expression between the LH and NLH lines. The conclusion from the work presented here is that the family of genes thus selected would be ideal candidate genes for linkage studies in human populations.

REFERENCES

Adrien, J., Dugovic, C., & Martin, P. (1991). Sleep-wakefulness patterns in the helpless rat. *Physiology and Behavior, 49,* 257–262.

Asberg, M., Traskman, L., & Thoren, P. (1976). 5-HIAA in the cerebrospinal fluid: A biochemical suicide predictor? *Archives of General Psychiatry 33,* 1193–1197.

Edwards, E., Harkins, K., Wright, G., & Henn, F. (1991). Modulation of [^{3}H] paroxetine binding to the 5HT uptake site in an animal model of depression. *Journal of Neurochemistry, 56,* 1581–1586.

Edwards, E., Harkins, K., Wright, G., & Henn, F. (1990). Effects of bilateral adrenalectomy on the induction of learned helplessness behavior. *Neuropsychopharmacology, 3,* 109–114.

Edwards, E., Muneyyirci, J., van Houten, P., Michel, C., & Henn, F. A. (1991). Opioid mechanisms in rats bred for learned helplessness. Social for Neuroscience 21st annual meeting, #322.11, p. 813.

Greenberg, L., Edwards, E., & Henn, F. A. (1989). Dexamethasone suppression test in helpless rats. *Biological Psychiatry, 26,* 165–168.

Gross-Isseroff, R., Salma, D. Israeli, M., & Biegon, A. (1989). Autoradiographic analysis of tritiated imipramine binding in the human brain post mortem: Effects of suicide. *Archives of General Psychiatry 46,* 237–241.

Gross-Isseroff, R., Dillon, K. A., Israeli, M., & Biegon, A. (1990). Regionally selective increases in μ-opioid receptor density in brains of suicide victims. *Brain Research, 530,* 312–316.

Henn, F. A., Johnson, J., Edwards, E., & Anderson, D. (1985). Melancholia in rodents: Neurobiology and pharmacology. *Psychopharmacology Bulletin, 21*, 443–446.

Janowsky, R., Okada, F., Manier, D., Applegate, C. D., & Sulser, F. (1982). Role of serotonergic input in the regulation of the β adrenergic receptor coupled adenylate cyclase system. *Science, 218*, 990–991.

Leshner, A. I., & Segal, M. (1979). Fornix transection blocks "learned helplessness" in rats. *Behavioral and Neural Biology, 26*, 497–501.

Linnoila, M., Virkkunen, M., Scheinin, M., Nuuitila, A., Rimon, R., & Goodwin, F. K. (1983). Low cerebrospinal fluid 5-HIAA concentration differentiates impulsive from nonimpulsive violent behavior. *Life Science, 33*, 2609–2614.

Mann, J. J., Stanley, M., McBride, P. A., & McEwen, B. (1986). Increased serotonin and β-adrenergic receptor binding in the frontal cortices of suicide victims. *Archives of General Psychiatry, 43*, 954–959.

Martin, J. V., Edwards, E., Johnson, J. O., & Henn, F. A. (1990). Monoamine receptors in an animal model of affective disorders. *Journal of Neurochemistry, 55*, 1142–1148.

Mishra, R., Janowsky, A., & Sulser, F. (1980). Action of mianserin and zemelidine on norepinephrine receptor coupled adenylate cyclase system in brain: subsensitivity without reduction in α-2 noradrenergic receptor binding. *Neuropharmacology, 19*, 983–989.

Overmeier, J. B., & Seligman, M. E. P. (1967). Effects of inescapable shock upon subsequent escape and avoidance responding. *Journal of Comparative Physiology Psychology, 63*, 28.

Papez, J. W. (1937). A proposed mechanism of emotion. *Archives of Neurological Psychiatry, 38*, 725–743.

Sachar, E., Hellman, L., Roffwag, H. P., Halpern, F. S., Fukushima, D. K., & Gallagher, T. F. (1973). Disrupted 24-hour cortisol secretion in psychotic depression. *Archives General Psychiatry, 28*, 19–26.

Sapolsky, R., & Plotsky, P. (1990). Hypercortisolism and its possible neural basis. *Biology Psychiatry, 27*, 937–952.

Simson, P. G., Weiss, J. M., Hoffman, L. J., & Ambrose, M. J. (1986). Reversal of behavioral depression by infusion of an α_2 agonist into the locus coeruleus. *Neuropharmacology, 25*, 385–389.

Sorensen, S., Palmer, M. R., Dunwiddie, T., & Hoffer, B. (1980). Electrophysiological correlates of ethanol induced sedation in differentially sensitive lines of mice. *Science, 210*, 1143–1145.

Stockmeier, C. A., Martino, A. M., & Kellar, K. J. (1985). A strong influence of serotonin axons on β-adrenergic receptors in rat brain. *Science, 230*, 323–325.

Weiss, J. M., Goodman, P. A., Losito, B. B., Corrigan, S., Charry, J. M., & Bailey, W. H. (1981). Behavioral depression produced by an uncontrollable stressor: Relationship to norepinephrine, dopamine and serotonin levels in various regions of rat brain. *Brain Research Review, 3,* 167–205.

Weiss, J. M., Goodman, P. A., & Bailey, W. H. (1982). A model for neurochemical study of depression in behavioral models and the analysis of drug action. *Proceedings, 27th OHOLO Conference,* Zichron Ya'acov, Israel, pp. 195–223.

Young, E. A., Murphy-Weinberg, R. F. V., Haskett, S. S., Watson, S., & Akil, H. (1991) Loss of glucocorticoid fast feedback in depression. *Archives of General Psychiatry, 48,* 693–699.

10

Lithium's Effect on Gene Expression
Implications for the Pathogenesis of Mood Disorders

HERBERT M. LACHMAN

Despite years of clinical experience and volumes of published basic research, the molecular basis of lithium's therapeutic action in the treatment of manic-depressive illness is not well understood. When one considers lithium's relative simplicity (it is number 3 on the atomic table of elements), the inability to explain its mechanism of action becomes more enigmatic. It is believed by many investigators that understanding its mechanism of action may provide insight into the molecular and genetic basis of manic-depressive illness, similar to the hypothesis that dopaminergic pathways are involved in the pathogenesis of schizophrenia, which is based on the physiological action of neuroleptics. On the other hand, the therapeutic efficacy of many pharmacological agents may have little to do with pathogenesis. After all, how much would be understood about coronary artery disease if the extent of our knowledge about this condition were limited to the observation that calcium channel blockers and β-receptor antagonists were effective treatments? Nevertheless, considering the problems associated with using linkage analysis in studying the genetics of mood

---

The Program in Behavioral Genetics is supported by the Ruane Family Fund and the G. Harold and Leila Y. Mathers charitable foundation. The author is a fellow of the Irma T. Hirschl and Monique Weill-Caulier charitable trust. He would like to thank Dr. Herman van Praag for his encouragement and support in establishing the program.

disorders, as discussed elsewhere in this text, and the relative inaccessibility of the human brain to experimental manipulation, studying the basis of lithium's action appears to be a valid experimental approach.

Lithium salts were introduced into medical practice in the 1850s as a treatment for gout and rheumatoid arthritis. The discovery of their antimanic effect in the late 1940s was made by serendipity. John Cade, an Australian psychiatrist, observed that guinea pigs were sedated with lithium carbonate and reasoned that this property could be exploited in patients with manic psychosis (Cade, 1949). Although the reasoning was faulty as strong sedatives are not necessarily effective antimanic agents, the drug indeed had a dramatic clinical debut. Furthermore, Cade's experimental observation in guinea pigs was fortuitous since lithium sedates rodents at toxic concentrations and does not cause significant sedation in humans. Therefore, the findings that led to the first clinical trial of lithium in manic-depressive patients were based on an incorrect conclusion drawn from an aberrant experimental observation.

The widespread utilization of the drug was delayed for several years because of the reports of severe toxicity and death associated with its use. Noack and Trautner (1951) showed that toxicity was related to high serum lithium levels and that a therapeutic effect could be safely secured with careful monitoring. One wonders whether this remarkable drug would even be considered for use now if it were introduced for the first time in today's litigious society.

Since the earliest use of lithium in the late 1940s, a number of theories have been proposed to explain the mechanism of its antimanic action. These have largely reflected popular biological themes of specific research eras. Cade (1949) originally suggested that abnormal urate metabolism played a role in the development of manic psychosis and that the increased solubility of lithium urate as compared with the sodium salt was responsible for the antimanic effect. This hypothesis represents a 1950s' perspective that emphasized metabolic pathways. Later, with the emergence of the "catecholamine hypothesis," attempts were made to understand lithium's action based on its effect on norepinephrine metabolism and adrenergic-coupled neuronal events (Belmaker, 1981). More recently, lithium's influence on cholinergic, dopaminergic, and serotonergic pathways became a focus of investigation as the importance of these systems in regulating limbic system activity was recognized (Belmaker, 1981; Pert, Rosenblatt, Sivit, Pert, & Bunney, 1978). One problem in determining the precise molecular site of lithium's action based on its overall effect on a particular neurotransmitter pathway is that the interactive nature of neuronal systems in the central nervous system (CNS) makes it difficult to differentiate between direct and indirect effects. One way to attempt to simplify the study of a drug's action is to perform experiments in cultured neuronal cell lines. In this experimental system, one can more easily manipulate cellular responses, using well-characterized pharmacological agents, without considering the indirect effects of interactive neurotransmitter pathways. Furthermore, in cell lines one can focus more directly on specific biochemical pathways by using inhibitors or activators that may be difficult to use in whole animals because of toxicity or the lack of brain-blood barrier penetrance.

Based on the use of relatively simple biological systems such as cultured neuronal cell lines and cell-free systems, newer theories concerning the molecular basis of lithium's action have emerged that suggest an inhibitory effect on intracellular signal transduction and second-messenger synthesis. These hypotheses are not mutually exclusive of lithium's putative effects on major neurotransmitter systems since the actions of norepinephrine, serotonin, dopamine, and acetylcholine are, to a large extent, mediated by signal transduction pathways. This chapter reviews the effect of lithium on signal transduction and shows how it led to our investigation of a novel site of lithium action—at the level of second messenger-mediated gene expression.

SIGNAL TRANSDUCTION

Signal transduction is a generic term used to describe cellular communication and the intracellular transfer of biological information. The activation of signal transduction pathways following exposure to ligands present in the extracellular space, such as hormones, growth factors, and neurotransmitters, results in the synthesis of second messengers and the activation of a cascade of intracellular events leading to functional changes in the cell. With the exception of glucocorticoids and several other hormones, ligands bind to membrane-anchored receptors and do not enter the cell.

Neurotransmitter binding may lead directly to the opening of an ion channel, a situation that occurs when the receptor itself is a "ligand-activated" channel, such as the nicotinic cholinergic receptor (Greenberg, 1989). Alternatively, a number of neurotransmitter and neuropeptide receptors function by activating or inhibiting the synthesis of intracellular second messengers (Berridge & Irvine, 1989; Nishizuka, 1986; Gilman, 1989; Spiegel, 1987) (Figure 10–1). Since ligands of this type do not enter the cell, the second messengers serve to

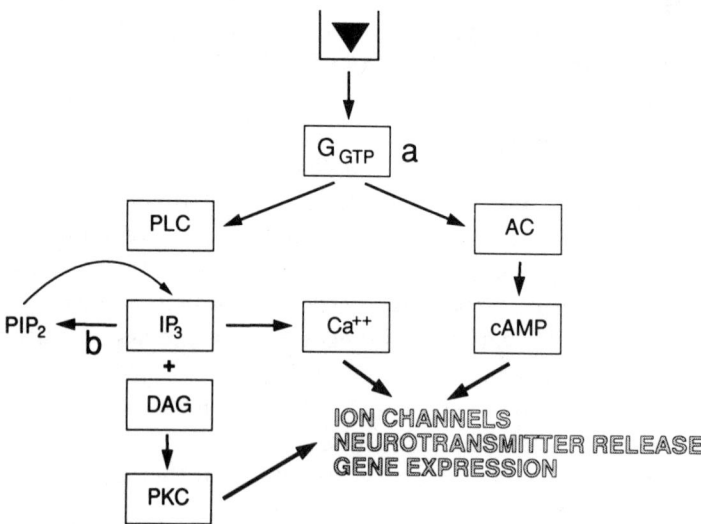

Figure 10–1. Signal transduction and putative sites of lithium action. Signal transduction is initiated by ligand (inverted filled triangle) binding to specific receptors. This leads to G-protein activation (G_{GTP}), which, in turn, stimulates one of several second-messenger systems. The two shown are adenylate cyclase (AC), which results in the transient accumulation of cAMP, and phospholipase C (PLC), which catalyzes the hydrolysis of the membrane phospholipid PIP_2 into inositol 1,4,5-trisphosphate (IP_3) and diacylglycerol (DAG) (different G proteins are coupled to these two signal transduction pathways). IP_3 mobilizes Ca^{2+}, whereas DAG activates the serine phosphorylase protein kinase C (PKC). PKC, cAMP, and Ca^{2+} regulate a variety of effector targets. Two proposed sites of lithium action are inhibition of G proteins (site a) and inhibition of myoinositol 1-phosphatase, which is involved in recycling IP_3 into inositol and ultimately PIP_2 (site b).

"transduce" the signal generated by receptor activation. Second messengers influence a wide variety of intracellular responses, including neurotransmitter release, ion channel conductivity, and receptor function. Depending on the receptor system, the same neurotransmitter may open a ligand-gated ion channel or couple to an intracellular second-messenger system. For example, acetylcholine may bind to either the nicotinic receptor or one of several muscarinic receptor subtypes that regulate second-messenger synthesis (Goyal, 1989).

LITHIUM AND THE PHOSPHOINOSITIDE PATHWAY

The signal transduction pathways implicated as targets of lithium's action in neuronal cells include the phosphoinositide (PI) and G-protein–coupled pathways (Sherman, Leavitt, Honchar, Hallchar, & Phillips, 1981; Berridge & Irvine, 1989; Lachman & Papolos, 1989; Newman & Belmaker, 1987). The basic scheme of the PI pathway is that certain receptors, such as the serotonin (5-HT$_{1c}$) and the M$_1$ muscarinic receptors, are linked to the activation of a membrane-bound enzyme, phospholipase C (PLC). This enzyme cleaves the membrane phospholipid phosphatidyl inositol 4,5-bisphosphate (PIP$_2$) to generate the second messengers IP$_3$, which mobilizes Ca^{2+} (Berridge & Irvine, 1989), and diacylglycerol, which activates protein kinase C (PKC) (Nishizuka, 1986, 1989). PKC plays an important role in signal transduction since it phosphorylates serine residues on a number of target proteins involved in regulating cell growth and neuronal transmission (Nishizuka, 1989). The IP$_3$ is rapidly dephosphorylated by several phosphatase enzymes into inositol phosphate (IP) intermediates that are recycled into inositol, and ultimately PIP$_2$ (see Figure 10–1). Allison and Stewart (1971) found that lithium is a potent noncompetitive inhibitor of myoinositol 1-phosphatase (M1P), a critical enzyme in the inositol recycling pathway. Michael Berridge, who was awarded the 1989 Lasker award for his work on the discovery of IP$_3$, and others have proposed that the inhibition of M1P could result in a decrease in neuronal inositol and PIP$_2$, an effect termed the "inositol depletion hypothesis." In this model, manic-depressive illness could be due to an increase in PI-mediated neuronal responses that are attenuated by lithium's inhibition of PIP_2 (Berridge & Irvine, 1989; Hallcher & Sherman, 1980; Lachman & Papolos, 1989). This hypothesis is attractive for three reasons: (1) The selective action of lithium in patients with mood disorders compared with its lack of effect on the mood of normal individuals could be explained by the noncompetitive nature of MIP inhibition, which would be more readily observed in a pathologically overactive PI pathway. (2) Since the brain–blood barrier is impermeable to free serum inositol, neuronal cells would be expected to exhibit increased susceptibility to inositol depletion by lithium, consistent with its relatively selective neuronal action at therapeutic concentrations. (3) It is consistent with the delay that occurs in lithium's therapeutic effect since PIP_2 depletion would take place only after the PIP_2 pool synthesized prior to lithium treatment was exhausted.

Experimental support for the inositol-depletion hypothesis comes from studies demonstrating reduced brain phosphoinositide turnover and PIP_2 levels in rats treated chronically with lithium (Elphick, Taghavi, Powell, & Godfrey, 1988; Sherman, Leavitt, Honchar, Hallcher, & Phillips, 1981). It has also been shown that lithium inhibits hippocampal cholinergic responses coupled to PLC, an effect observed only following excessive cholinergic stimulation (Worley, Heller, Snyder, & Baraban, 1988). According to the inositol-depletion hypothesis, repetitive agonist stimulation would be required to deplete the pool of PIP_2 established prior to lithium blockade.

LITHIUM AND ITS EFFECT ON G PROTEINS

It has also been suggested by a number of investigators that lithium inhibits G proteins (Avissar, Schreiber, Danon, & Belmaker, 1988; Belmaker, 1981; Newman & Belmaker, 1987). These proteins are critical mediators of signal transduction pathways since they couple receptors to second-messenger activation and inhibition. G proteins, located on the inner surface of cell membranes, are closely coupled to receptors. Following ligand stimulation, G proteins bind a molecule of guanoine triphosphate (GTP) and activate a cascade of intracellular events leading to the stimulation or inhibition of various second-messenger systems and effector targets. Included among its actions are regulation of PLC, adenylate cyclase, phospholipase A2, and potassium channel conductivity (Axelrod, Burch, & Jelsema, 1988; Gilman, 1989; Ross, 1989; Spiegel, 1987).

In membrane preparations, agonists promote GTP binding, an effect attributed to G-protein activation. It has been shown that therapeutic concentrations of lithium potently inhibit this response (Mark & Geisler, 1989). This is consistent with cellular studies demonstrating that lithium inhibits agonist-stimulated cyclic adenosine monophosphate (cAMP) accumulation, which is thought to be due to an effect at the level of G_s, the G protein coupled to adenylate cyclase (Newman & Belmaker, 1987). One side effect of lithium treatment, vasopressin-resistant nephrogenic diabetes insipidus, may be due to the inhibition of vasopressin-stimulated adenylate cyclase in renal tubules.

SECOND MESSENGER-MEDIATED GENE EXPRESSION

As alluded to previously, the PI and cAMP pathways are coupled to a variety of electrophysiological events that lead to relatively rapid changes in neuronal responses. An emerging area of interest in the neurosciences is understanding the mechanism by which short-term changes in neuronal activity may lead to more long-term effects on neuronal function. Long-term changes are required to explain such phenomena as learning, conditioned responses, and memory storage. It is also conceivable that long-term changes should be considered in the pathogenesis of mood disorders since an acute stressful event may initiate a depressive episode that lasts many months. Second messenger systems appear to play an important role in long-term neuronal events through the regulation of gene expression and synaptic plasticity.

Gene expression refers to all of the events leading to the accumulation of a messenger RNA (mRNA) in the cytoplasm. These include gene transcription, during which a precursor RNA copy of a gene is made; RNA splicing and processing; polyadenylation; and cytoplasmic transport. One of the most fascinating and still evolving stories of modern biology has been the elucidation of the mechanisms involved in the regulation of gene expression. Unfortunately, a detailed discussion is not within the scope of this text, but a number of excellent reviews written by the investigators primarily responsible for these fundamental discoveries are available (Sharp, 1989; Ptashne, 1988, 1989). This discussion will be limited to the aspects of gene regulation related to lithium's effects on second-messenger–mediated gene expression.

Genes are transcribed into RNA by a complex group of specific and nonspecific proteins. The nonspecific factors include such enzymes as RNA polymerase II, which binds to the so-called promoter region located in front (the 5' region) of virtually every gene. RNA polymerase II, in combination with other factors, initiates and directs the synthesis of RNA from a DNA template. The DNA binding site for these transcription factors is essentially the same for most genes. Specific factors involved in regulating gene expression include proteins that bind to DNA elements found only near subsets of genes. These factors play an important role in cellular differentiation and tissue-specific gene expression.

In addition to factors that initiate or enhance gene expression, a number of genes are also regulated by factors that inhibit expression. These could include proteins that bind to DNA and cause local conformational changes that prevent RNA polymerase II binding. Alternatively, some proteins inhibit gene expression by binding to and inhibiting proteins that ordinarily would enhance transcription (Diamond, Miner, Yoshinaga, & Yamamoto, 1990; Schule et al., 1990; Yang-Yen et al., 1990).

Another aspect of gene expression pertinent to this discussion is the operational difference between constitutive and inducible gene expression. The term constitutive refers to gene expression that occurs at a basal, steady-state level, whereas inducible expression is the burst of transcriptional activation (or inhibition) that takes place following stimulation by agonists such as hormones, growth factors, or neuromodulators. Genes that are expressed constitutively may also retain the capacity for inducible expression as well. For example, a number of genes encoding neuropeptides, such as neuropeptide Y (NPY), are expressed at high basal levels, yet are capable of severalfold increases following stimulation by modulators that increase the transcription factors that bind to the NPY gene.

The PI and cAMP pathways are both coupled to the regulation of gene expression. Induction of cAMP-dependent kinase leads to the activation of a cAMP-responsive element binding protein (CREB) that binds to specific DNA sequences referred to as CRE (cAMP-responsive element) to stimulate gene transcription (Comb et al., 1988; Mellon, Clegg, Cornell, & McKnight, 1989; Sassone-Corsi, Visvader, Ferland, Mellon, & Verma, 1988). Induction of the PI pathway leads to PKC activation, which modulates gene expression by activating proteins that bind to so-called phorbol ester or tumor-promoter–responsive (TRE) DNA elements. An important target of both PKC and cAMP is the *fos* proto-oncogene, which encodes a protein that forms a dimer with the product of the *jun* gene (Comb et al., 1988; Curran & Teich, 1982; Greenberg, Ziff, & Greene, 1986; Rauscher et al., 1988a,b; Sheng & Greenberg, 1990). The Fos/Jun heterodimer, along with the dimers formed between closely related Fos and Jun-like proteins, forms a family of transcription factors that are referred to as AP-1. Consequently, regulation of *fos* expression leads to changes in the expression of a multitude of genes that contain AP-1 binding domains. Since a number of genes expressed in the CNS are regulated by PKC, cAMP, and AP-1, the pathway that leads from synaptic release of neuromodulators to gene expression is critical in understanding normal neuronal function.

EFFECT OF LITHIUM ON GENE EXPRESSION IN CULTURED NEURONAL CELLS

Because of the effect of the PI and cAMP signal transduction pathways on transcription regulation, we reasoned that lithium would have an inhibitory effect on *fos* gene expression. Our first experiments were performed on the PC12 rat pheochromocytoma cell line. The experimental protocol essentially involved extracting RNA from cells treated with agonists that stimulate either the cAMP or PI pathway, in the presence or absence of lithium. Furthermore, these pathways were also stimulated by drugs that directly activate second-messenger synthesis and, therefore, bypass the receptor–G-protein portion of the signal transduction pathway. These drugs included the phorbol ester phorbol 12-myristate 13-acetate (PMA) and forskolin, which directly stimulate PKC and adenylate cyclase respectively.

The RNA was analyzed by gel electrophoresis and Northern filter hybridization. In this technique, equal aliquots of RNA are separated by electrophoresis through a denaturing gel. This resolves RNA molecules by size, with the smaller fragments migrating more rapidly than the larger fragments. The RNA is then transferred to an RNA binding filter and hybridized with single-stranded, radioactive-labeled copies of genes of interest. In this experiment, *fos* and a control gene encoding glyceraldehyde phosphate dehydrogenase (GAPDH) were used. A radioactive signal is generated on x-ray film when the complementary strand of the radioactive probe binds to the specific mRNA. The signal intensity is proportional to the relative level of mRNA present in the cells. As seen in Figure 10–2, *fos* mRNA is not detected in unstimulated PC12 cells, whereas hybridization with the control gene results in a relatively strong GAPDH mRNA signal. However, upon treatment with carbachol, a stable but nonspecific cholinergic agonist, a large increase in *fos* mRNA was detected after 30 minutes. Pretreatment with pirenzepine, a muscarinic antagonist with relative M1 receptor specificity, results in marked *fos* signal attenuation. This

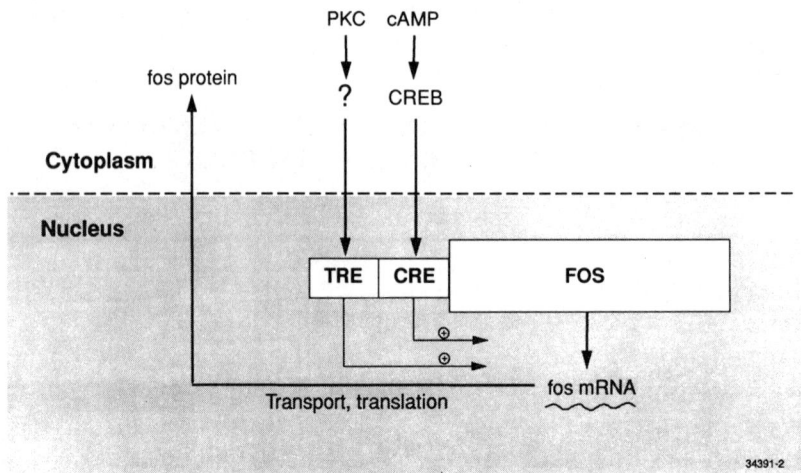

Figure 10–2. Regulation of *fos* gene expression. PKC and cAMP activate factors that bind to DNA regulatory elements located in front of the *fos* gene. Undefined factors activated by PKC bind to the TRE (tumor-promoter-responsive) DNA element. Cyclic AMP-dependent kinase activates a cAMP-responsive element binding protein (CREB) that binds to the CRE region of the gene. Both events lead to activation of *fos* gene transcription and the synthesis of *fos* messenger RNA (mRNA). The mRNA is transported to the cytoplasm, where it is translated into Fos protein.

suggests that in the PC12 subclone used in our experiments, induction of *fos* mRNA by carbachol is mediated by the M1 receptor subtype, which is coupled to the PI pathway and activation of PKC.

An unexpected experimental result was observed when the cells were pretreated with lithium chloride for two to 16 hours prior to carbachol stimulation. Although lithium alone did not significantly influence basal levels of *fos* mRNA, it caused a 10-fold enhancement of the carbachol stimulated *fos* mRNA signal (Kalasapudi, Sheftel, Divish, Papolos, & Lachman, 1990). This rapid effect of lithium on gene expression contrasts with the latency of its clinical antimanic action, a point that will be addressed later in this chapter. A similar enhancing effect was observed when the cells were stimulated with other PLC-coupled agonists, including bradykinin and nerve growth factor. In addition, an augmenting effect of lithium on *fos* expression has also been observed in U937 cells, a human monocytic leukemia cell line, although it was not detected in C6 glioma cells. By contrast, lithium had no effect on *fos* mRNA induced in PC12 cells by the cAMP activators forskolin and PGE_1, which activate adenylate cyclase directly or through a G-protein–coupled receptor respectively (Divish et al., 1991).

Initially, we felt that the lithium augmenting effect on *fos* mRNA was not necessarily inconsistent with its putative inhibition of inositol phospholipid metabolism. A fairly well-established experimental finding is that inhibition of M1P leads to the rapid accumulation of IP intermediates in lithium-treated cells exposed to agonists that stimulate PLC (Van Calker, Assmann, & Greil, 1987; Volonte, Parries, & Racker, 1988). Changes in the concentration of IP intermediates could conceivably alter the balance between IP isomers that increase Ca^{2+} mobilization and those that do not, especially with respect to the generation of $1,3,5\text{-}IP_3$, an IP intermediate that has a more prolonged effect on C^{2+} mobilization as compared with the $1,3,4IP_3$ isomer. Since *fos* expression is influenced by Ca^{2+} through the activation of calmodulin kinase, or through PKC, which is a Ca^{2+}-dependent enzyme, it is conceivable that an alteration in the ratio of bioactive IP intermediates could lead to rapid changes in *fos* expression.

To determine whether this could be a mechanism of lithium's effect on gene expression, we induced *fos* mRNA by treating PC12 cells with

PMA to activate PKC directly. Since phorbol esters bypass the putative site of lithium's action in the PI cycle, cells treated with this class of compounds do not accumulate IP intermediates. We found that similar to receptor-mediated agonists, lithium-enhanced PMA induced *fos* expression. These data suggested to us that lithium acts at a novel site in the PI pathway, through enhancement of *fos* expression at the level of PKC-*fos* coupling. However, it is not clear at this time whether the effect is due to a direct action on PKC or results from its effect on a PKC-activated intermediate in the PKC-*fos* coupling pathway. This is an important distinction since enhancement at the PKC level would suggest that additional PKC targets may also be enhanced by the drug. The finding by Casebolt and Jope (1991) that lithium influences protein phosphorylation in hippocampal slices treated with phorbol esters suggests a direct effect on PKC.

EFFECT OF LITHIUM ON *fos* EXPRESSION IN RAT BRAIN

With the exception of muscarinic cholinergic induction of *fos*, which was observed using 1 mM of lithium, the augmenting effect in cell lines was most readily observed using relatively high concentrations of lithium (10 mM). Therefore, we were interested in determining whether a similar effect on *fos* expression could be detected in the brain using nontoxic concentrations. The analysis of *fos* expression in the brain is a novel experimental strategy used by molecular neurobiologists to demonstrate neuronal activation. Curran and Morgan (1985) were the first to demonstrate that neurophysiological events are coupled to gene expression. Since then, a number of investigators have clearly shown that *fos* mRNA and Fos protein are activated by neuronal activity induced in the CNS. For example, *fos* mRNA accumulates in the hippocampus following electrical and drug-induced seizures (Davis, Nakajima, Gleiter, Post, & Marangos, 1989). In addition, exposure to environmental light and sensory stimulation induces *fos* expression in the superchiasmatic nucleus and spinal sensory tracts respectively (Kornhauser, Nelson, Mayo, & Takahashi, 1990; Toele, Castro-Lopez, Coimbra, & Zieglegansberger, 1990).

However, *fos* expression induced in the brain by cholinergic stimulation had not been previously reported.

In one experiment, rats were treated with pilocarpine, a centrally active muscarinic agonist or vehicle. Although basal levels of *fos* mRNA are quite low in the brain, we detected a substantial increase in the cortex, and to a lesser extent, in the hippocampus, 75 minutes after pilocarpine treatment. Although the brain is a rich source of several muscarinic receptor subtypes, the induction of *fos* mRNA by pilocarpine appears to be primarily mediated by the M1 subtype since it was substantially inhibited by pirenzepine. In order to determine the effect of lithium on *fos* expression, we treated two groups of rats with a single intraperitoneal injection of lithium (3 meq/kg) or an equimolar dose of sodium chloride. Seven hours later, the rats were treated with pilocarpine and sacrificed after 75 minutes. To control for equal loading and transfer of the RNA, we analyzed *fos* mRNA in comparison with a constitutively expressed control gene that encodes the mitochondrial enzyme malate dehydrogenase (MDH). The RNA data were quantitated by densitometric analysis and the *fos*/MDH mRNA ratio determined. We found that lithium-enhanced pilocarpine induced *fos* expression by 2.7-fold compared with sodium-chloride and pilocarpine-treated controls (Figure 10–3), similar to the effect observed in PC12 cells. The serum lithium level at the time of sacrifice ranged between 0.45 and 0.81, which is within the therapeutic range in patients with mood disorders. Lithium chloride alone did not appreciably increase basal *fos* mRNA in the cortex or hippocampus. An enhancing effect was also observed in pilocarpine-treated rats administered lithium chloride for five days. In contrast to these findings, induction of *fos* mRNA using a single electroconvulsive shock was neither enhanced nor inhibited by lithium, which suggests that the effect is relatively specific.

These data are similar to the reports by other investigators who have described lithium augmentation of central cholinergic function (Lerer & Stanley, 1985; Levy, Zohar, & Belmaker, 1983). The relatively selective effect on pilocarpine-induced *fos* expression in the brain and the sensitivity of the M1 muscarinic system in PC12 cells to lithium are consistent with an antimanic effect according to the cholinergic

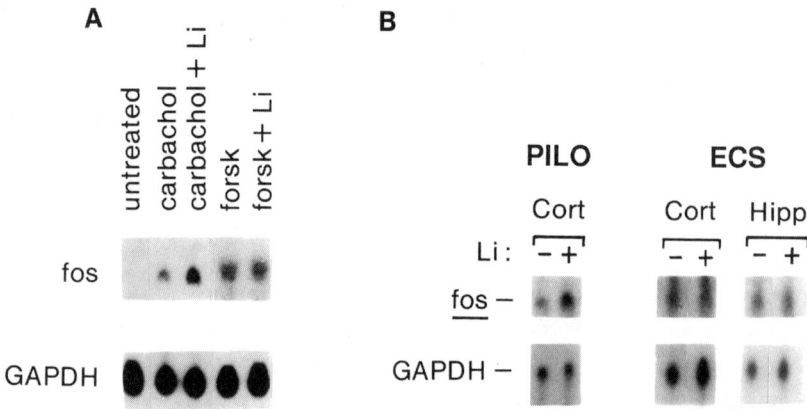

Figure 10–3. Effect of lithium on gene expression. (A.) RNA was extracted from PC12 pheochromocytoma cells and analyzed for *fos* mRNA and a control mRNA encoding the enzyme GAPDH (glyceraldehyde phosphate dehydrogenase) using Northern hybridization analysis. Cells were treated with carbachol, a cholinergic agonist, and forskolin, an inducer of adenylate cyclase, in the presence and absence of lithium chloride (10 mM). The autoradiographic signals how a substantial increase in carbachol-induced *fos* mRNA in the presence of lithium. Induction of *fos* mRNA by carbachol is blocked by pirenzepine, a relatively selective M1 muscarinic antagonist (data not shown). (B.) RNA was extracted from the cortex of rats 75 minutes after treatment with pilocarpine. Rats were pretreated seven hours earlier with 1.5 meq/kg lithium chloride administered by intraperitonial injection (+) or an equimolar quantity of sodium chloride (−). RNA was extracted from the cortex and hippocampus 75 minutes after a single electroconvulsive inducing shock. In this experiment, lithium specifically enhanced pilocarpine-induced *fos* mRNA 2.5-fold. Similar results were obtained in the cumulative analysis involving seven rats ($p < 0.05$) (densitometric and cumulative data not shown).

hypothesis—a premise that suggests that mania is due to reduced cholinergic drive (Janowsky, Risch, Parker, Huey, & Judd, 1980; Dilsaver, 1986).

EFFECT OF LITHIUM ON NEUROPEPTIDE GENE EXPRESSION

It could be argued that the effect of lithium on rats treated with high doses of a pharmacological agent such as pilocarpine may not closely reproduce conditions that are found in patients with manic-depressive illness. Therefore, it was of interest to examine the effect of lithium on gene expression in the brain under more basal physiological conditions. The *fos* gene is a poor marker for this type of analysis since its basal expression is quite low. Therefore, as target genes, we chose neuropeptide Y (NPY) and preproenkephalin (enk), both of which are expressed at relatively high levels in a number of brain regions, including the hippocampus, cortex, and hypothalamus. NPY, a 36-amino-acid peptide, is, in fact, the most abundant peptide in the brain (Tatemoto, Carlquist, & Mutt, 1982). These neuropeptides are also of interest because of the important behavioral effects observed following their central administration, which include regulation of the hypothalamic-pituitary axis (HPA), increased feeding behavior, and alteration of circadian rhythms (Albers & Ferris, 1984; Inui, Inoue, & Nakajima, 1991; Levine & Morley, 1984). Enk has an effect on the reward and motivation systems (Belluzzi & Stein, 1977). The effect of NPY on feeding may be particularly relevant since it is a potent inducer of carbohydrate feeding in rats and carbohydrate craving is found in patients with atypical depression, the most common form of depression in patients with bipolar disorder. Also, the dysregulation of the HPA and the phase shifting of circadian rhythms that occur in patients with mood disorders suggest that NPY, as well as other peptides, may be involved in the pathogenesis of mood disorders (Wahlestedt, Ekman, & Widerlov, 1989; Widerlov, Lindstrom, Wahlestedt, & Ekman, 1988).

NPY and enk gene expression are regulated by the second-messenger systems implicated as targets of lithium's action. In cell lines, NPY is expressed constitutively and is also induced by activators of PKC and cAMP (Higuchi, Yang, & Sobol, 1988). Similarly, the 5' promoter region of the enk gene contains phorbol-ester–responsive and cAMP-responsive DNA elements (Comb et al., 1988; Van Nguyen, Kobierski, Comb, & Hyman, 1990).

In order to determine the effect of lithium on genes that encode neuropeptides, the kinetics of cytosolic mRNA accumulation had to be taken into account. In the *fos* experiments, RNA was extracted one-half to two hours after agonist stimulation because *fos* mRNA has a very short half-life (approximately 10 minutes). Consequently, *fos* mRNA accumulates rapidly after transcriptional activation and disappears within a few hours. Although agonist-stimulated transcription of NPY and enk is also quite rapid, the mRNAs exhibit a slower turnover rate and, therefore, accumulate more slowly in the cytosol. In cell lines, enk mRNA increases over a period of 4 to 8 hours after stimulation, whereas NPY requires 24 to 48 hours (Comb et al., 1988; Higuchi et al., 1988; Sonnenberg, Rauscher, Morgan, & Curran, 1989). In order to explore the effect of short-term lithium treatment on neuropeptide gene expression, the following experiment was performed. Rats were treated with a single intraperitoneal injection of either lithium or sodium chloride between 8 A.M. and 9 A.M. (1.5 meq/kg). Twelve hours later, a second injection was administered, and the animals were sacrificed the following morning. We found that lithium-treated rats exhibited a statistically significant 40% increase in the NPY/MDH mRNA ratio as compared with sodium-chloride–treated controls ($n = 6$, $p < 0.05$). In contrast, we did not observe any significant change in the enk/MDH mRNA ratio (Figure 10–4).

Since enk mRNA accumulates four to eight hours after agonist stimulation in cell cultures, and with a similar time course in the brain following electroconvulsive shock, we also studied the effect of lithium on enk mRNA eight hours after a single intraperitoneal lithium injection. Although there was approximately a 20% decrease in the enk/MDH ratio in lithium-treated rats as compared with those treated with an equimolar amount of sodium chloride, the results were not statistically significant ($n = 6$, $p > 0.2$). These data suggest that the lithium-enhancing effect on hippocampal NPY expression is relatively selective.

Another reason why NPY was chosen as a target gene for investigation is its capacity for induction by glucocorticoids (GC). NPY mRNA is increased in PC12 cells treated with dexamethasone, a synthetic GC, and decreases in the arcuate nucleus following adrenalectomy (Higuchi et al., 1988; White, Dean, & Martin, 1990). These events are probably mediated by a GCH receptor–responsive-like element located in the first intron of the NPY gene. The rationale for studying GC-mediated gene expression in the brain is based on interesting clinical observations in humans and behavioral studies in animals. When used in clinical practice, GCs such as prednisone induce feelings of euphoria and have been found to precipitate manic and depressive episodes

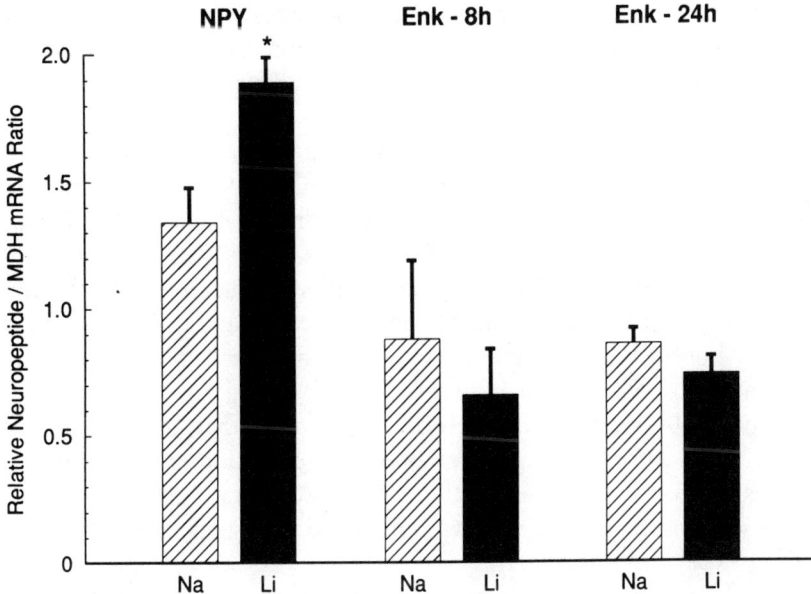

Figure 10–4. Effect of lithium on neuropeptide Y (NPY) and pre-proenkephalin (enk) gene expression. Nine rats were treated with 1.5 meq/kg lithium chloride or sodium chloide (intraperitonial) twice in a 24-hour period. RNA was extracted from the hippocampus and analyzed for NPY and enk mRNA. In addition, the RNA was analyzed with a gene-encoding malate dehydrogenase (MDH) which was used as a control. The autoradiographic signals were quantitated by densitometry, and the NPY/MDH and enk/MDH ratios were calculated. In addition, the enk/MDH ratio was calculated for samples obtained eight hours after a single intraperitonial injection of lithium or sodium chloride ($N = 6$ in each group). The increase in the NPY/MDH ratio induced by lithium is significant using a student's T-test ($p < 0.05$, $N = 9$).

in bipolar individuals (Wolkowitz et al., 1990). Indeed, one study demonstrated that lithium may provide prophylaxis against GC-induced psychosis (Falk, Mahnke, & Poskanzer, 1979).

Glucocorticoids also have an effect in animal models of depression. Fritz Henn and others have developed a model in rats based on a learned helpless paradigm (see Chapter 9). Henn and co-workers have shown that the development of learned helplessness can markedly enhanced by adrenalectomy, which removes the endogenous source of GCs (Edwards, Harkins, Wright, & Henn, 1990). The presence of abundant (GR) GC receptors in the limbic system, especially the hippocampus, suggests that this is the anatomical site that mediates the effects of GCs on mood (McEwen, DeKloet, & Rostene, 1986; McEwen et al., 1990).

On a molecular level, GC functions, in part, by regulating gene expression (Reul & DeKloet, 1985; Yamamoto, 1985). A soluble GR found in the cytosol is transformed into a transcription factor following steroid binding. Activated GRs have the capacity to enhance or inhibit gene expression, depending on a number of factors, including cell type, the presence of other transcription factors, and the nature of the GR-responsive element (GRE) found in the gene's promoter region (Yamamoto, 1985; Diamond et al., 1990).

These observations have led us to postulate that certain patients with mood disorders may have abnormal regulation of GC-regulated genes in the CNS. Consequently, lithium's effect on gene expression, in particular, its influence on GC-mediated genes, appears to be a relevant experimental concern.

In the rat hippocampus, we were able to detect a 40% increase in the NPY/MDH mRNA ratio 24 hours after a single intraperitoneal injection of corticosterone acetate (CA) (compared with vehicle-injected rats). This increase in very similar to that afforded by lithium. When multiple agents independently increase gene expression, their combination often results in additive or synergistic activation. Consequently, the effect of combined CA and lithium treatment on NPY expression was determined. We found that the NPY/MDH mRNA ratio was not significantly different in CA- and lithium-treated rats as compared with CA- and sodium-chloride–treated controls. This result suggests that lithium and GCs may partially attenuate their respective capacities fully to induce NPY gene expression in the hippocampus, an effect opposite to that found by Dobner Tischler, Lee, Bloom, and Donahue (1988), who showed that lithium-enhanced dexamethasone induced neurotensin/neuromedin N-gene expression in PC12 cells.

Although these findings are preliminary and must be confirmed for other GC-induced genes, it is interesting to speculate on a possible mechanism. One possibility is that GRs and a lithium-activated transcription factor are interfering with their respective capacities to induce NPY gene expression. This type of negative interaction has recently been reported to occur between GR and AP-1 (Diamond et al., 1990; Schule et al., 1990; Yang-Yen et al., 1990). Regardless of the mechanism, a moderating effect of lithium on GC-induced gene expression would be consistent with the hypothesis that abnormal GC responses in the brain are important in the pathogenesis of mood disorders.

CONCLUSIONS

We believe that lithium's effect on gene expression represents a novel target of its action in neuronal cells. Our results are consistent with the mRNA enhancement detected in lithium cell lines and in rat brain described by several investigators (Arenander, de Vellis, & Herschman, 1989; Dobner et al., 1988; Sivam, Strunk, Smith, & Hong, 1986; Sivam et al., 1989). Although the precise mechanism of this effect has not been clearly elucidated, it does not appear that previous concepts of lithium's action adequately explain the phenomenon. The inositol-depletion hypothesis is not consistent with the observed effects since one would expect inhibition of PI-mediated gene expression to occur and not augmentation. In addition, inositol depletion is consistent neither with the time course of the lithium-enhancing effect, which occurs within one to two hours, nor with the observation that *fos* expression induced by phorbol esters, which bypass the phosphoinositide cycle, is augmented by lithium.

Similarly, the effect is not consistent with lithium's putative inhibition of G proteins since one would expect a reduction in either PLC or G-protein/adenylate cyclase–mediated gene expression, and no effect using phorbol esters, which also bypass G-proteins. As described earlier, the data are most consistent with a novel enhancing effect occurring at the level of PKC-*fos* coupling.

At this time, we can only speculate on the possible clinical relevance of these findings. One immediate concern is the time course of the observed changes in gene expression, which is measured in hours, compared with the latency required to observe a clinical antimanic effect with lithium. Although the delayed therapeutic action is consistent with the inositol-depletion hypothesis, it is not necessarily inconsistent with the rapid effect on gene expression. One possibility is that the underlying physiological and neuroendocrine abnormalities responsible for the manic state exhibit a long-half-life, measured in days or weeks. Consequently, lithium could rapidly increase the expression of a set of target genes that are underexpressed in manic individuals, but a clinical effect would not be realized until the factors responsible for the manic behavior had undergone an appropriate loss of activity. Another possibility is that the target genes induced by lithium may not exert a rapid effect on neuronal activity because of an inherent delay between gene activation and a physiological effect of the encoded protein. For example, the delay in translating and processing a preneuropeptide mRNA into protein and then transporting the protein to the nerve terminal could account for a considerable amount of time.

The antidepressant action of lithium may be more consistent with the gene expression scenario. Lithium has been found to augment tricyclic antidepressants in patients who have only had a partial therapeutic response (Heninger, Charney, & Sternberg, 1983), an effect that is usually observed within 24 to 48 hours. Accordingly, a gene product that is reduced in depressed individuals, and that may be required for an adequate response to tricyclics, may be rapidly enhanced by lithium. It is interesting to note that several investigators have found that NPY levels are reduced in the cerebrospinal fluid of patients with depression (Widerlov et al., 1988). It has been suggested that some of the behavioral and endocrine changes exhibited by patients with mood disorders could be due to abnormal neuropeptide expression within limbic structures. Consequently, lithium's rapid and selective enhancement of NPY gene expression may be directly related to an antidepressant effect according to this model.

A number of the stressors that influence mood in patients with depression and manic-depressive illness appear to function by regulating gene expression. Glucocorticoids were discussed earlier, but estrogens, progesterones, and thyroid hormone all can influence mood and exert their physiological effect, in part, by regulating gene expression. Similar to GC, these hormones bind to cytosolic receptors that are transformed into transcription factors (Bradley, Young, & Weinberger, 1989; Brown & Sharp, 1990). Consequently, since lithium influences gene expression, a further analysis of its effect on endocrine and pharmacological stressors that influence mood, and on a molecular level modulate gene expression, may be an interesting experimental approach to understanding the molecular basis of manic-depressive illness.

REFERENCES

Albers, H. E., & Ferris, C. F. (1984). Neuropeptide Y: Role in light–dark cycle entrainment of hamster circadian rhythms. *Neuroscience Letters, 50*, 163–168.

Allison, J. H., & Stewart, M. A. (1971). Reduced brain inositol in lithium treated rats. *Nature, 233*, 267–268.

Arenander, A. T., de Vellis, J., & Herschman, H. R. (1989). Induction of c-fos and TIS genes in cultured rat astrocytes by neurotransmitters. *Journal of Neuroscience Research, 24*, 107–114.

Avissar, S., Schreiber, G., Danon, A., & Belmaker, R. H. (1988). Lithium inhibits adrenergic and cholinergic increases in GTP binding in rat cortex. *Nature, 331*, 440–442.

Axelrod, J., Burch, R. M., & Jelsema, C. L. (1988). Receptor mediated action of phospholipase A2 via GTP-binding proteins: Arachidonic acid and its metabolites as second messengers. *Trends in Neurosciences, 11* (3), 117–123.

Belluzzi, J. D., & Stein, L. (1977). Enkephalin may mediate euphoria and drive-reduction reward. *Nature, 266*, 556–558.

Belmaker, R. H. (1981). Receptors, adenylate cyclase, depression and lithium. *Biological Psychiatry, 16* (4), 333–349.

Berridge, M. J., & Irvine, R. F. (1989). Inositol phophates and cell signalling. *Nature, 341*, 197–205.

Bradley, O. J., Young, W. S., & Weinberger, C. (1989). Differential expression of alpha and beta thyroid receptor genes in rat brain and pituitary. *Proceedings of the National Academy of Sciences, 86* (16), 2250–2254.

Brown, M., & Sharp, P. A. (1990). Human estrogen receptor forms multiple protein-DNA complexes. *Journal of Biological Chemistry, 265* (19), 11238–11243.

Cade, J. F. J. (1949). Lithium salts in the treatment of psychotic excitement. *Medical Journal Australia, 2*, 349–352.

Casebolt, T. L., & Jope, R. S. (1991). Effects of chronic lithium treatment on protein kinase C and cyclic AMP dependent protein phosphorylation. *Biological Psychiatry, 29*, 233–243.

Comb, M., Mermond, N., Hyman, S. E., Pearlberg, J., Ross, M. E., & Goodman, H. M. (1988). Proteins bound at adjacent DNA elements act synergistically to regulate human proenkephalin cAMP inducible transcription. *EMBO Journal, 7,* 3793–3805.

Curran, T., & Morgan, J. I. (1985). Superinduction of C-fos by nerve growth factor in the presence of peripherally active benzodiazepines. *Science, 229,* 1265–1268.

Curran, T., & Teich, N. M. (1982). Candidate product of the FBJ murine osteosarcoma virus oncogene: Characterization of a 55,000 dalton phosphoprotein. *Journal of Virology, 42,* 114–122.

Davis, J. L., Nakajima, T., Gleiter, C. H., Post, R. M., & Marangos, P. J. (1989). Mouse brain C-fos MRNA distribution following a single electroconvulsive shock. *Journal of Neurochemistry, 52,* 1954–1957.

Diamond, M. I., Miner, J. N., Yoshinaga, S. K., & Yamamoto, K. R. (1990). Transcription factor interactions: Selectors of positive or negative regulation from a single DNA element. *Science, 249,* 1266–1272.

Dilsaver, S. C. (1986). Cholinergic mechanisms in depression. *Brain Research Reviews, 11,* 285–316.

Divish, M. M., Sheftel, G., Boyle, A., Kalasapudi, V. D., Papolos, D. F., & Lachman, H. M. (1991). Differential effect of lithium on fos protooncogene expression mediated by receptor and post-receptor activators of protein kinase C and cyclic adenosine monophosphate: Model for its antimanic action. *Journal of Neuroscience Research, 28,* 40–48.

Dobner, P. R., Tischler, A. S., Lee, Y. C., Bloom, S. R., & Donahue, S. R. (1988). Lithium dramatically potentiates neurotensin/neuromedin N-gene expression. *Journal of Biological Chemistry, 263,* 13983–13986.

Edwards, E., Harkins, K., Wright, G., & Henn, F. (1990). Effects of bilateral adrenalectomy on the induction of learned helpless behavior. *Neuropsychopharmacology, 3,* 109–114.

Elphick, M., Taghavi, Z., Powell, T., & Godfrey, P. P. (1988). Alteration of inositol phospholipid metabolism in rat cortex by lithium but not carbamazepine. *European Journal of Pharmacology, 156,* 411–414.

Falk, W. E., Mahnke, M. W., & Poskanzer, D. C. (1979). Lithium prophylaxis of corticotropin-induced psychosis. *Journal of the American Medical Association, 241,* 1011–1012.

Gilman, A. G. (1989). G-proteins and regulation of adenylate cyclase. *Journal of the American Medical Association, 13,* 1819–1825.

Goyal, R. (1989). Muscarinic receptor subtypes. *New England Journal of Medicine, 321* (15), 1022–1029.

Greenberg, D. (1989). Calcium channels and calcium channel agonists. *Annals of Neurology, 21,* 317–330.

Greenberg, M. E., Ziff, E. B., & Greene, L. A. (1986). Stimulation of neuronal acetylreceptors induces rapid gene transcription. *Science, 234,* 80–83.

Hallcher, L., & Sherman, W. R. (1980). The effects of lithium ion and other agents on the activity of myo-inositol-1-phosphatase from bovine brain. *Journal of Biological Chemistry, 261,* 8100–8130.

Heninger, G. R., Charney, D. S., & Sternberg, D. E. (1983). Lithium potentiation of antidepressant treatment. *Archives of General Psychiatry, 40,* 1335–1342.

Higuchi, H., Yang, H. Y. T., & Sobol, S. (1988). Rat neuropeptide Y precursor gene expression. *Journal of Biology Chemistry, 262,* 6288–6295.

Inui, A., Inoue, T., & Nakajima, M. (1991). Brain neuropeptide Y in the control of adrenocorticotropic hormone secretion in the dog. *Brain Research, 510,* 211–215.

Janowsky, D. S., Risch, S. C., Parker, D., Huey, L. Y., & Judd, L. (1980). Increased vulnerability to cholinergic stimulation in affective disorder patients. *Psychopharmacology Bulletin, 16,* 29–31.

Kalasapudi, V. D., Sheftel, G., Divish, M. M., Papolos, D. F., & Lachman, H. M. (1990). Lithium augments fos protooncogene expression in PC12 pheochromocytoma cells: Implications for therapeutic action of lithium. *Brain Research, 521,* 47–54.

Kornhauser, J. M., Nelson, D., Mayo, K. E., & Takahashi, J. S. (1990). Photic and circadian regulation of C-fos gene expression in the hamster superchiasmatic nucleus. *Neuron, 5,* 127–134.

Lachman, H. M., & Papolos, D. F. (1989). Abnormal signal transduction: A hypothetical model for bipolar affective disorder. *Life Sciences, 45,* 1413–1426.

Lerer, B., & Stanley, M. (1985). Effect of lithium on cholinergic mediated responses and [^{3}H] QNB binding in rat brain. *Brain Research, 344,* 211–219.

Levine, A. S., & Morley, J. E. (1984). Neuropeptide Y (NPY). A potent inducer of consummatory behavior in rats. *Peptides, 5,* 1025–1028.

Levy, A., Zohar, J., & Belmaker, R. H. (1983). The effect of chronic lithium pretreatment on rat brain muscarinic receptor regulation. *Neuropsychopharmacology, 21,* 1199–1201.

McEwen, B. S., DeKloet, E. R., Rostene, W. (1986). Adrenal steroid receptors and actions in the nervous system. *Physiology Review, 66,* 1121–1188.

McEwen, S., Brinton, P. E., Chao, H. M., Coirini, H., Gannon, M. N., Gould, E., O'Callaghan, J., Spencer, R., Sakai, R., & Willey, C. (1990). The hippocampus: A site for moderating interactions between steroid hormones, neurotransmitters, and neuropeptides. In E. C. Mulle & R. M. McCloud (Eds.), *Neuroendocrine perspective* (Vol. 8, pp. 93–131). New York: Springer-Verlag.

Mellon, P. L., Clegg, C., Cornell, L.A., & McKnight, G. S. (1989). Regulation of transcription by cAMP-dependent protein kinase. *Proceedings of the National Academy of Sciences, 86,* 488–491.

Mark, A., & Geisler, A. (1989). Effects of GTP on hormone-stimulated adenylate cyclase in cerebral cortex, striatum, and hippocampus from rats treated chronically with lithium. *Biological Psychiatry, 26,* 279–288.

Newman, M. E., & Belmaker, R. H. (1987). Effects of lithium in vitro and ex vivo on components of the adenylcyclase system in membranes from cerebral cortex of the rat. *Neuropharmacology, 26,* 211–217.

Nishizuka, Y. (1986). Studies and perspectives of protein kinase C. *Science, 233,* 305–312.

Nishizuka, Y. (1989). The family of protein kinase C for signal transduction. *Journal of the American Medical Association, 13,* 1826–1833.

Noack, H., & Trautner, E. M. (1951). Lithium treatment of maniacal psychosis. *Medical Journal of Australia, 21,* 219–222.

Pert, A., Rosenblatt, J. E., Sivit, C., Pert, C. B., & Bunney, W. E. (1978). Long term treatment with lithium prevents the development of dopamine receptor sensitivity. *Science, 201,* 171–173.

Ptashne, M. (1988). How eukaryotic transcription factors work. *Nature, 335,* 683–689.

Ptashne, M. (1989). How gene activators work. *Scientific American, 260* (1), 40–47.

Rauscher, F. J., Cohen, D. R., Curran, T., Bos, T. J., Vogt, P. K., Bohmann, D., Tijan, R., & Franza, R. (1988a). Fos-associated protein p39 is the product of the jun proto-oncogene. *Science, 240,* 1010–1016.

Rauscher, F. J., Sambucetti, L. C., Curran, T., Distel, R. J., & Spiegalman, B. M. (1988b). Common DNA binding site for fos protein complexes and transcription factor AP-1. *Cell, 52,* 471–480.

Reul, J. M. H. M., & DeKloet, E. R. (1985). Two receptor systems for corticosterone in rat brain: Microdistribution and differential occupation. *Endocrinology, 97,* 223–230.

Ross, E. M. (1989). Signal sorting and amplification through G-protein coupled receptors. *Neuron, 3,* 141–152.

Sassone-Corsi, P., Visvader, J., Ferland, L., Mellon, P. L., & Verma, I. M. (1988). Induction of proto-oncogene fos transcription through the adenylate cyclase pathway: Characterization of a c-AMP responsive element. *Genes and Development, 2,* 1529–1538.

Schule, R., Rangarajan, P., Kliewer, S., Ransone, L. J., Bolado, J., Yang, N., Verma, I. M., & Evans, R. M. (1990). Functional antagonism between oncoprotein C-jun and the glucocorticoid receptor. *Cell, 62*, 1217–1226.

Sharp, P. A. (1989). Gene regulation and oncogenes. *Cancer Research, 49* (8), 2188–2194.

Sheng, M., & Greenberg, M. (1990). The regulation and function of C-fos and other immediate early genes in the nervous system. *Neuron, 4*, 477–485.

Sherman, W. R., Leavitt, A. L., Honchar, M. P., Hallcher, L., & Phillips, B. E. (1981). Evidence that lithium alters phosphoinositide metabolism: Chronic administration elevates primarily D-myo-inositol-1-phosphate in cerebral cortex of the rat. *Journal of Neurochemistry, 36* (6), 1947–1951.

Sivam, S. P., Krause, J. E., Takeuchi, K., Li, S., McGinyy, J. F., & Hong, J. S. (1989). Lithium increases rat striatal beta and gamma preprotachykinin messenger RNAs. *Journal of Pharmacology and Experimental Therapeutics, 248*, 1297–1301.

Sivam, S. P., Strunk, C., Smith, D. R., & Hong, J. S. (1986). Proenkephalin-A gene regulation in the rat striatum: Influence of lithium and haloperidol. *Molecular Pharmacology, 30*, 186–191.

Sonnenberg, J. L., Rauscher, F. J., Morgan, J. I., & Curran, T. (1989). Regulation of proenkephalin by fos and jun. *Science, 246*, 1622–1625.

Spiegel, A. M. (1987). Signal transduction by guanine nucleotide binding proteins. *Molecular and Cellular Endocrinology, 49*, 1–16.

Tatemoto, K., Carlquist, M., & Mutt, V. (1982). Neuropeptide Y: A novel brain peptide with structural similarities to peptide YY and pancreatic polypeptide. *Nature, 296*, 659–660.

Toele, T. R., Castro-Lopez, J. M., Coimbra, A., & Ziegleganzberger, W. (1990). Opiates modify induction of C-fos protooncogene in the spinal cord of the rat following noxious stimulation. *Neuroscience Letters, 111*, 46–51.

Van Calker, D., Assmann, K., Greil, W. (1987). Stimulation by bradykinin, angiotensin 2, and carbachol of the accumulation of inositol phosphates in PC12 pheochromocytoma cells: Differential effects of lithium on mono and polyphosphates. *Journal of Neurochemistry, 49*, 1379–1384.

Van Nguyen, T., Kobierski, L., Comb, M., & Hyman, S. E. (1990). The effect of depolarization on expression of the human proenkephalin gene is synergistic with cAMP and dependent upon a cAMP inducible enhancer. *Journal of Neuroscience, 10* (8), 2825–2833.

Volonte, C., Parries, G. S., & Racker, E. (1988). Stimulation of inosital incorporation into lipids of PCIZ cells by nerve growth factor and bradykinin. *Journal of Neurochemistry, 51,* 1156–1162.

Wahlestedt, C., Ekman, R., & Widerlov, E. (1989). Neuropeptide Y and the central nervous system: Distribution and possible relationship to neurological and psychiatric disorders. *Progress in Neuropsychopharmacology & Biological Psychiatry, 13,* 31–54.

White, B. D., Dean, R., & Martin, R. J. (1990). Adrenalectomy decreases neuropeptide Y mRNA levels in the arcuate nucleus. *Brain Research Bulletin, 25,* 711–715.

Widerlov, E., Lindstrom, L. H., Wahlestedt, L., & Ekman, R. (1988). Neuropeptide Y and peptide YY as possible cerebrospinal fluid markers for major depression and schizophrenia respectively. *Journal of Psychiatric Research, 22,* 22–26.

Wolkowitz, O. M., Rubinow, D., Doran, A. R., Breier, A., Berrettini, W. H., Kling, M. A., & Pickar, D. (1990). Prednisone effects on neurochemistry and behavior. *Archives of General Psychiatry, 47,* 963–968.

Worley, P. F., Heller, W. A., Snyder, S. H., & Baraban, J. M. (1988). Lithium blocks a phosphoinositide-mediated cholinergic response in hippocampal slices. *Science, 239,* 1428–1429.

Yamamoto, K. R. (1985). Steroid receptor regulated transcription of specific genes and gene networks. *Annual Reviewing Genetics, 19,* 209–252.

Yang-Yen, H. F., Chambard, J. C., Sun, Y. L., Smeal, T., Schmidt, T. J., Drouin, J., & Karin, M. (1990). Transcriptional interference between C-jun and the glucocorticoid receptor: Mutual inhibition of DNA binding due to direct protein-protein interaction. *Cell, 62,* 1205–1215.

Author Index

Adland, M. L., 122, 154
Adrian, C., 121, 122, 154
Adrien, J., 179
Akil, H., 183
Akiskal, H. S., 121, 127, 150, 154, 161
Akots, G., 65
Albers, H. E., 207
Allen, C. R., 33, 73, 78, 83, 87, 88, 92, 101, 109, 149
Allen, M. G., 15
Allison, J. H., 197
Altis, D., 33, 39
Altshuler, K. Z., 151, 152
Ambrose, M. J., 181
Anderson, C. M., 33, 128, 130, 149
Anderson, D., 178
Anderson, M. A., 65
Anderson, S., 92, 109
Andreasen, N. C., 7, 10, 11, 31, 32, 43, 44, 101, 123, 125, 139, 150, 153, 159
Angst, J., 75, 124, 153
Applegate, C. D., 187
Ardlean, V., 140
Arenander, A. T., 211
Asberg, M., 181
Assmann, K., 203
Avissar, S., 198
Axelrod, J., 199

Baastrup, P. C., 124
Babron, M. C., 109
Bailey, J., 88
Bailey, W. H., 178, 179
Baille, D., 92
Baldessarini, R. J., 126, 139
Bale, S. J., 85, 86, 101, 109, 149
Baltimore, D., 49

Baraban, J. M., 198
Baren, M., 17
Barker, D., 65
Barker, J. B., 105
Barnard E. A., 110
Barnard, P. J., 110
Baron, M., 10, 36, 92, 106, 107, 111, 148, 149, 151, 152, 155, 159
Barraclough, B., 92
Bateson, A. N., 110
Bazzoui, W., 74
Beardslee, W. R., 121
Bech, P., 107
Belluzzi, J. D., 207
Belmaker, R. H., 36, 92, 106, 111, 148, 194, 195, 197, 198, 199, 205
Bemporad, J., 121
Benieralcis, C., 143
Berg, B., 147
Berman, R., 143
Berrettini, H., 149
Berrettini, W. H., 47, 66, 92, 109, 110, 140, 149, 209
Berridge, M. J., 196, 197, 198
Bertelsen, A., 13, 15, 120
Betelson, C. J., 46
Biederman, J., 150
Biegon, A., 185, 189
Birley, J. L. T., 140
Bishop, D. S., 129, 130
Bishop, J. M., 46
Blackwood, D., 92, 109
Bland, S. D., 87, 92, 101
Blazer, D. B., 152
Bloom, S. R., 210, 211
Bocchetta, A., 106, 107
Bohmann, D., 201

Bolado, J., 200, 211
Bolstein, D., 108
Bonaiti-Pellie, C., 98
Bonilla, E., 65
Boorman, D., 92, 109, 149
Bos, T. J., 201
Botstein, D., 61
Boularand, S., 109
Boyd, J. H., 120
Boyle, A., 203
Bradley, O. J., 212
Braman, J. C., 65
Breier, A., 209
Brinton, P. E., 210
Brocas, H., 92, 110
Brody, G. H., 140
Brown, G. W., 140
Brown, M., 212
Brown, R. J., 108
Brown, V., 65
Bruell, J. H., 17
Brynjolfsson, J., 92, 109
Buchanan, J. A., 46, 65
Buchwald, M., 46, 65
Buckle, V. J., 110
Bunney, W. E., 31, 66, 150, 151, 152, 195
Bunney, W. E., Jr., 10, 106, 107
Burch, R. M., 199
Burge, D., 121, 122, 154
Burke, J. D., Jr., 6, 7
Burney, E., 121
Burroughs, J., 125
Byck, R., 33

Cade, J. F. J., 194
Cadoret, R. J., 17, 18
Campbell, J., 149
Campion, D., 109
Cantwell, D. P., 17
Cappellari, C. B., 47
Carlquist, M., 207
Carlson, G., 124
Carney, M. W. P., 162
Carothers, A., 109
Carre-Pigeon, F., 110
Carter, A. S., 122, 154
Caruso, M. A., 110
Casebolt, T. L., 204

Castiglione, C. M., 82, 92
Castro-Lopez, J. M., 204
Cavalli-Sforza, L. L., 92
Chakravarti, A., 46, 65, 109, 111
Chambard, J. C., 200, 210
Chao, H. M., 210
Chapman, C. J., 6
Charney, D. S., 212
Charon, F., 92, 110
Charry, J. M., 178
Christodorescu, D., 140
Clayton, P. J., 106
Clayton, P., 10, 31, 32
Clegg, C., 201
Clerget-Darpoux, F., 98, 106, 109
Clifford, C. A., 15
Cochran, S. D., 140
Cohen, D. R., 201
Coimbra, A., 204
Coirini, H., 210
Cole, G. L., 46, 65
Collett-Feener, C. A., 46
Collins, F. S., 46, 65
Comb, M., 201, 207, 208
Cones, C., 128
Conneally, P. M., 65
Conte, G., 85, 86, 101, 109, 149
Cooklin, R. S., 162
Correll, L.A., 201
Corrigan, S., 178
Corsini, G. U., 106, 107
Coryell, W., 10, 11, 31, 32, 33, 39, 101, 126, 139, 150, 159
Cox, T. K., 46, 65
Coyne, J. C., 129
Cramer, G., 66
Crick, F. H. C., 48
Croughan, J., 44
Crouse, J., 106
Crowe, R. R., 10, 108, 109, 111, 149
Cummings, E. M., 122, 154
Curran, T., 201, 204, 208
Cytryn, L., 123, 154

Danforth, H., 125
Danon, A., 198
Darlison, M. G., 110
Darnell, J., 49

Author Index 221

Davenport, Y. B., 122, 154, 166
Davis, J. L., 204
Davis, J., 66
Davis, R. W., 61, 108
de Miguel, C., 92
de Vellis, J., 211
Dean, M., 46, 65
Dean, R., 208
Decina, P., 121
DeKloet, E. R., 210
Del Zompo, M., 106, 107
Denise, E., 109
Derrz, J., 110
Des Lauriers, A., 109
Detera-Wadleigh, S. D., 92, 109, 110, 149
Detera-Wadleigh, S., 149
Detre, T., 33
Deutsch, C. K., 17
Diamond, M. I., 200, 210, 211
Dibble, E. D., 149, 166
Dibble, E., 6, 10, 31, 150, 151, 152
Dillon, K. A., 185, 189
Dilsaver, S. C., 66, 206
Distel, R. J., 201
Divish, M. M., 203
Dobbs, M., 92
Dobner, P. R., 210, 211
Donahue, S. R., 210, 211
Donald, J., 109
Donis-Keller, H., 65
Doran, A. R., 209
Dougherty, D., 121
Downs, J., 121
Dozy, A. M., 82
Drouin, J., 200, 210
Drumer, D., 92, 148
Drumm, M., 46, 65
Dudleston, K., 92
Dugovic, C., 179
Dunner, D. L., 140
Dunwiddie, T., 188

Edwards, E., 178, 180, 181, 182, 183, 209
Egeland, J. A., 25, 33, 73, 74, 76, 77, 78, 82, 83, 85, 86, 87, 88, 92, 101, 109, 122, 149, 154, 160, 162
Eiberg, H., 65
Eisman, J., 109

Ekman, R., 207, 212
Elphick, M., 198
Elston, R. C., 19, 20, 108
Encio, I., 92
Endicott, J., 7, 10, 11, 31, 32, 33, 36, 39, 43, 44, 73, 92, 101, 111, 123, 125, 139, 150, 153, 159
Epstein, N. B., 129, 130
Eshleman, S. K., III, 160
Essen-Moller, E., 6
Evans, H. J., 92, 109
Evans, R. M., 200, 211

Falk, W. E., 209
Falloon, I. R. H., 129, 130
Falls, K., 88
Faraone, S. V., 4, 5, 6, 8, 14, 22, 120, 121, 123, 148, 149, 150, 151, 152, 153, 155, 159, 161, 162, 164, 168
Farber, S., 121
Fava, G. A., 164
Fawcett, J. A., 139
Feinberg, K. G., 147, 148, 161, 165
Feinberg, S. S., 147, 148, 154, 155, 157, 159, 161, 165, 166
Feinstein, C., 110
Feldman, D. M., 147
Felston, R. C., 111
Ferland, L., 201
Ferris, C. F., 207
Fieve, R. R., 106, 121
Fieve, R., 153
Filippi, G., 107
First, M. B., 43
Fischer, A., 7
Fishman, R., 7, 31, 32, 101, 123, 145, 153
Flanagan, S. D., 66
Fleiss J. L., 106, 111
Flood, C., 106
Florio, L. P., 152
Floris, G., 126
Forehand, R., 140
Frank, E., 109, 111, 128, 130, 143
Frankel, D. R., 109, 111
Franza, R., 201
Freeman, R., 125
Freeman, W. B., 129, 130
Fremming, G. H., 6

Friedman, S. L., 122
Fritsch, E. F., 53
Fritze, J., 109
Fruzzetti, A. E., 129, 130
Fujita, N., 110
Fukushima, D. K., 183
Fulker, D. W., 15

Gaensbauer, T. J., 154
Gallagher, T. F., 183
Gammon, G. D., 121
Gannon, M. N., 210
Gargan, M., 121
Gastpar, M., 107
Geisler, A., 199
Gejman, P. V., 149
Gelernter, J., 110, 149
Gerhard, D. S., 78, 82, 83, 85, 86, 87, 92, 101, 109, 149
Gerner, R. H., 129
Gershon, E. H., 47
Gershon, E. J., 106
Gershon, E. S., 6, 7, 10, 31, 66, 75, 92, 106, 107, 109, 110, 123, 125, 140, 149, 150, 151, 152, 155, 156, 161, 162, 163, 164, 166
Gesman, P. V., 110
Gheeysen, F., 109
Gibbon, M., 43
Gill, M., 109
Gilman, A. G., 196, 199
Ginns, E. I., 85, 86, 88, 101, 109, 149
Giuffra, L. A., 92
Glassner, B., 147
Gleiter, C. H., 204
Godfrey, P. P., 198
Goedken, R. J., 109, 111
Goeken, N., 149
Goetzl, V., 108
Gold, P. W., 122
Goldin, L. R., 10, 31, 92, 106, 107, 109, 110, 140, 149, 150, 151, 152
Goldsmith, B., 110
Goldstein, A. M., 85, 86, 101, 109, 149
Goldstein, M. J., 129
Goodman, A. B., 162
Goodman, H. M., 201, 207, 208
Goodman, P. A., 178, 179

Goodwin, F. K., 122, 126, 129, 154, 161, 181
Gordon, D., 122
Gordon, G., 154
Gosden, C., 109
Goshen-Gottstein, E. R., 147, 148
Gould, E., 210
Goyal, R., 197
Gravius, T., 65, 88
Green R., 108
Greenberg, D., 196
Greenberg, L., 183
Greenberg, M. E., 201
Greene, L. A., 201
Greil, W., 203
Grigoroiu-Serbanescu, M., 140
Grochweinski, V. J., 128
Grof, P., 124
Gross-Isseroff, R., 185, 189
Grove, W. M., 10, 11, 33, 39, 101, 150
Gruenberg, E., 6, 7
Grunblatt, J., 148
Gurling, H., 92, 109
Guroff, J. J., 6, 7, 10, 31, 106, 123, 125, 150, 151, 152
Gusella, J. F., 65
Guttorsmen, S. A., 106

Hagnell, O., 6, 7
Halbreich, U., 154
Hallcher, L., 197, 198
Halpern, F. S., 183
Hamburger, R., 36, 92, 106, 111, 148
Hammen, C., 121, 122, 154
Hamovit, J., 6, 7, 10, 123, 125, 150, 151, 152
Hamovit, S., 31
Harkins, K., 181, 182, 209
Harmon, R. J., 154
Harvald, B., 13, 15, 120
Haskett, S. S., 183
Hatfield, A. B., 142
Hauge, M., 13, 15, 120
Helgason, T., 6
Heller, W. A., 198
Hellman, L., 183
Helms, C., 65
Heltzer, J. E., 6, 7
Hendersen, S., 128

Henderson, A. S., 16
Heninger, G. R., 212
Henn, F. A., 178, 180, 181, 182, 183, 209
Henriksson, B., 109
Herschman, H. R., 211
Hetherington, E. M., 154
Heywood, E., 18
Hibbs, E., 123
Hidaka, N., 46, 65
Higuchi, H., 207, 208
Hill, E., 111
Himmelhoch, J., 33
Hinchcliffe, M., 128
Hiroto, D., 122
Hiroto, G., 154
Hirsch, D., 109, 110
Hirschfeld, R. M. A., 7, 31, 32, 101, 123, 125, 126, 153
Hochez, J., 98
Hodge, S. E., 94, 98
Hodgkinson, S., 92, 109
Hoehe, M. R., 66
Hoffer, A., 15
Hoffer, B., 188
Hoffman, L. J., 181
Hoffman, W. F., 154
Hogarty, G. F., 128, 130
Holzinger, K. J., 14
Holzman, P. S., 66
Honchar, M. P., 197, 198
Hong, J. S., 211
Hooper, D., 128
Hopper, J. L., 15
Hostetter, A. M., 25, 33, 73, 74, 78, 83, 87, 92, 101, 109, 149, 160, 162
Housman, D. E., 78, 82, 83, 85, 86, 92, 101, 109, 149
Hrubec, Z., 15
Hubbard, A., 92
Hudson, J. I., 150
Huey, L. Y., 66, 206
Hughes, H. B., 109, 111
Humphries, P., 109
Hyman, S. E., 201, 207, 208

Iannuzzi, M. C., 46, 65
Inoue, T., 207
Inui, A., 207

Irvine, R. F., 196, 197, 198
Israeli, M., 185, 189

Jackson, R., 108
Jaenicke, C., 122, 154
James, J. W., 14, 19
James, N. M., 6
Jamison, K. R., 127, 129, 154, 161
Janowsky, A., 185
Janowsky, D. S., 66, 206
Janowsky, R., 187
Jardine, R., 16
Jarrett, D. B., 128
Jelsema, C. L., 199
Jipescu, I., 140
John, K., 121
Johnson, J., 178, 180
Johnson, W. E., 124, 130, 139
Jones, S., 129, 130
Jope, R. S., 204
Jordan, P., 121
Jorna, T., 106, 123
Joy, V. D., 128
Joyce, P. R., 124, 131
Judd, L., 66, 206

Kalasapudi, V. D., 203
Kan, Y. W., 82
Kaplan, B. B., 109, 111
Karin, M., 200, 210
Karno, M., 152
Kaufmann, C. A., 146, 149, 169
Keenan, K., 150
Keisling, R., 127
Keith, T., 88
Keitner, G. I., 129, 130
Kellar, K. J., 187
Keller, M. B., 7, 33, 39, 121, 123, 125, 126, 139
Keller, M., 10, 31, 32, 139
Kellner, R., 164
Kelsoe, J. R., 85, 86, 101, 109, 149
Kennedy, D., 46, 65
Kennedy, J. L., 92
Kerem, B., 46, 65
Kestenbaum, C. J., 121
Kety, S. S., 18, 119, 121
Kidd, J. R., 82, 92

Kidd, K. K., 6, 10, 19, 77, 78, 82, 83, 85,
  86, 92, 94, 98, 101, 107, 109, 149
Kielholz, P., 107
King, S., 149
Klerman, G. L., 7, 31, 32, 101, 121, 123,
  125, 139, 153
Kliewer, S., 200, 211
Kling, M. A., 209
Knesevich, M. A., 39
Knowlton, R., 65
Kobierski, L., 207
Kochanska, G., 122
Körner, J., 109
Kornhauser, J. M., 204
Kraepelin, E. P., 153
Kramer, P. L., 82
Krause, J. E., 211
Kreisman, D. E., 128
Kremen, W. S., 22, 120
Kringlen, E., 66
Kron, L., 121
Kruger, S. D., 77, 107
Kuczynske, L., 122
Kukopulos, A., 126
Kunkel, L. M., 46
Kupfer, D. J., 29, 33, 109, 111, 124, 126,
  128, 130, 139, 143
Kurnit, D. M., 46
Kushner, S., 92, 106, 148
Kutcher, S., 153

LaBuda, M. C., 87, 92, 101
Lachman, H. M., 197, 198, 203
Lacy, L. G., 87, 92, 101
Laddomada, P., 126
Lampert, C., 125
Landolt, A. D., 143
Lange, K., 66
Lanke, J., 7
LaRoche, C., 143
Latte, B., 107
Lavori, P. W., 7, 123, 125, 126, 139
Leaf, P. J., 152
Leavitt, A. L., 197, 198
Lebo, R. V., 110
Leboyer, M., 109
Leckman, J. F., 6, 10, 31, 149, 150, 151, 152
Lee, Y. C., 210, 211

Legros, S., 92, 110
Leonhard, K., 143
Lepine, J. P., 109
Lerer, B., 205
Leshner, A. I., 182
Lester, E. P., 143
Levav, I., 162
Levin, S., 66
Levine, A. S., 207
Levitz, I. N., 147, 148
Levy, A., 205
Levy, D. L., 66
Li, S., 211
Liebman, C. S., 147
Liebowitz, J. H., 75, 162
Lin, S. P., 162
Lindstrom, L. H., 207, 212
Linkowski, P., 106, 107
Linnoila, M., 181
Lipinski, J. F., Jr., 124
Lipton, R. B., 66
Livingston Bruce, M., 152
Lodish, H., 49
Long, R. T., 85, 86, 88, 101, 109, 149
Losito, B. B., 178
Lunde, I., 18, 121

Mack, J. W., 153
Maclean, C. J., 149
Mahnke, M. W., 209
Maj, M., 143
Malafosse, A., 109
Mallet, J., 92, 109
Mallinger, A. G., 128
Mallya, G., 150, 161
Malzberg, B., 162
Mandel, B., 36, 92, 106, 111, 148
Maniatis, T., 53
Manier, D., 187
Mann, J. J., 184
Mansky, P. A., 124, 130, 139
Marangos, P. J., 204
Marchbanks, M., 109
Marchbanks, R., 92
Marinescu, E., 140
Markiewicz, D., 46, 65
Marrache, M., 143
Martin, J. B., 65

Martin, J. V., 180
Martin, N. G., 16
Martin, P., 179
Martin, R. J., 208
Martino, A. M., 187
Marton, P., 153
Mattheysse, S., 66
Matthyse, S., 106
Mayfield, A., 122, 154
Mayo, K. E., 204
McBride, P. A., 184
McCarthy, M. I., 109, 111
McDonald-Scott, P., 33, 39
McEachran, A. B., 128
McEwen, B., 184, 210
McEwen, S., 210
McGinniss, M. H., 149
McGinyy, J. F., 211
McInnis, M., 92, 109
McKeon, P., 109
McKnew, D., 122, 123, 154
McKnight, G. S., 201
Melica, A. M., 6, 9
Mellon, P. L., 201
Melmer, G., 46, 65
Mendlewicz, J., 17, 18, 92, 105, 106, 107, 108, 109, 110, 111, 120, 153
Merikangas, K. R., 29, 143, 161
Mermond, N., 201, 207, 208
Meselson, M., 50
Messner, K. H., 77
Michel, C., 181
Miklowitz, D. J., 129
Miller, I. W., 129, 130
Miner, J. N., 200, 210, 211
Mintz, J., 129
Mishra, R., 185
Mitchell, P., 109
Mohr, J., 65
Moises, H. W., 92
Molthan, L., 77
Moltz, D., 131
Monaro, A. P., 46
Morgan, J. I., 204, 208
Mork, A., 199
Morley, J. E., 207
Morrell, W., 125
Morris, C., 14, 19

Morrison, N., 109
Morton, L. A., 76, 82, 94, 98
Morton, N. E., 3, 6, 93, 149
Motulsky, A. G., 162
Muir, W., 92, 109
Muneyyirci, J., 181
Murphy-Weinberg, R. F. V., 183
Murray, R. M., 15
Mutt, V., 207
Myers, J. K., 6, 7

Nakajima, M., 207
Nakajima, T., 204
Namboodiri, K. K., 20
Naylor, S., 65
Nee, J., 10, 31, 32, 44
Negri, F., 6, 9
Neiswanger, K., 109, 111
Nelson, D., 204
Neve, R. L., 46
Newman, M. E., 197, 198, 199
Newman, M., 92, 106, 148
Nishizuka, Y., 196, 197
Noack, H., 194
Nuechterlein, K. H., 129
Nurnberger, H., 123, 125
Nurnberger, J. F., 31
Nurnberger, J. I., Jr., 7, 10, 140, 150, 151, 152, 153
Nuutila, A., 181

O'Callaghan, J., 210
O'Gorman, T. W., 18
O'Malley, K., 109
Offord, D. R., 73, 92, 101
Offord, R. D., 33
Ojesio, L., 7
Okada, F., 187
Olsen, T., 143
Olsson, K., 88
Ortmann, J., 18, 121
Orvaschel, H., 6, 7
Ott, J., 36, 93, 94, 111
Ottina, K., 65
Overmeier, J. B., 178

Pakstis, A. J., 82, 92
Palmer, D., 149

Palmer, M. R., 188
Palmer, P. J., 109, 111
Papez, J. W., 181
Papolos, D. F., 83, 129, 131, 132, 165, 197, 198, 203
Papolos, J., 83, 129, 165
Pardes, H., 146, 149, 169
Pare, C. M. B., 153
Parker, C., 65
Parker, D., 66, 206
Parri, J., 121
Parries, G. S., 203
Parsons, P. L., 6
Pascalis, G., 110
Paul, S. M., 85, 86, 88, 101, 109
Paul, S., 149
Pauls, D. C., 109, 122
Pauls, D. L., 6, 10, 33, 73, 76, 77, 78, 82, 83, 85, 86, 87, 88, 92, 101, 109, 149, 154
Pauls, D., 149
Pearlberg, J., 201, 207, 208
Pellegrini, D., 123
Penrose, L. S., 93
Perel, J. M., 128
Perris, C., 9, 108, 121
Persad, E., 106, 123
Pert, A., 195
Pert, C. B., 195
Petursson, H., 92, 109
Pfohl, B., 149
Phillips, B. E., 197, 198
Phipps, P., 88
Pickar, D., 209
Pincus, H. A., 146, 149, 169
Plavsic, N., 65
Pletcher, B. A., 82
Plonim, R., 154
Plotsky, P., 183
Pollin, W., 15
Pollitzer, W. S., 108
Pope, H. G., 124
Pope, H. G., Jr., 150
Popper, M., 162
Poskanzer, D. C., 209
Post, R. M., 124, 204
Potter, M., 92
Powell, T., 198
Prange, A., 108

Price, J., 151
Prien, R. F., 124, 126, 130, 139
Propping, P., 109
Pruitt, D. B., 121
Prusoff, B. A., 6, 10, 121, 128, 129, 130, 143
Ptashne, M., 200
Pyeritz, R. E., 162

Racker, E., 203
Radke-Yarrow, M., 122, 154
Rafaelsen, O. J., 107
Raffaele, P., 143
Rahav, M., 162
Rainer, J., 17, 18, 105, 108, 120
Rangarajan, P., 200, 211
Ransone, L. J., 200, 211
Rauscher, F. J., 201, 208
Ravindran, A., 162
Rediker, K., 65
Reeders, S., 92, 109
Regier, D. A., 6, 7
Reginaldi, D., 126
Reich, T., 7, 10, 11, 14, 19, 31, 32, 93, 101, 106, 123, 125, 150, 153, 159
Reiss, A. L., 110
Reiss, D. J., 128, 130
Reiss, D., 154
Reul, J. M. H. M., 210
Rice, J. P., 32, 33, 39, 106, 123
Rice, J., 7, 10, 11, 31, 32, 39, 93, 101, 123, 125, 126, 150, 153, 159
Rimon, R., 181
Riordan, J. R., 46, 65
Risch, N., 36, 92, 106, 107, 111, 148
Risch, S. C., 66, 206
Roberts, E. J., 128
Robins, E., 43, 73, 143, 159
Robins, L. N., 6, 7
Rochberg, N. J., 39
Roffwag, H. P., 183
Rogenline, N., 106
Rommens, J. M., 46, 65
Rorsman, B., 7
Rosenbaum, K., 110
Rosenblatt, J. E., 195
Rosenthal, D., 18, 119, 121
Ross, E. M., 199
Ross, M. E., 201, 207, 208

Rostene, W., 210
Rounsaville, B. J., 128, 129, 130
Rozmabel, R., 46, 65
Rubinow, D., 209
Ryder-Cook, A. S., 110

Sachar, E., 183
Sackeim, H. A., 121
Sakaguchi, A. Y., 65
Sakai, R., 210
Salma, D. 185
Sambrook, J., 53
Sambucetti, L. C., 201
Samolyk, D., 109
Sandkuyl, L. A., 36, 111
Sapolsky, R., 183
Sassone-Corsi, P., 201
Sceery, W., 10, 31, 150, 151, 152
Scheiner, R., 143
Scheinin, M., 181
Schindler, R., 163
Schlesser, M. A., 151, 152
Schmidt, T. J., 200, 210
Schofield, P. R., 110
Schou, M., 124, 126, 139
Schreiber, G., 198
Schreiber, J., 123
Schule, R., 200, 211
Schulsinger, F., 18, 121
Schulz, S. C., 152, 161, 164, 166
Schumm, J. W., 65
Schwab, J. J., 33, 73, 92, 101
Schwartzburg, M., 33
Seeburg, P. H., 110
Segal, M., 182
Seligman, M. E. P., 178
Serra, G., 126
Sevy, S., 92, 109, 110
Sharp, P. A., 200, 212
Shaw, M. W., 169
Sheftel, G., 203
Sheng, M., 201
Sherman, W. R., 197, 198
Sherrington, R., 92, 109
Shields, J., 15
Shine, J., 109
Shoulson, I., 65
Simon, P., 92, 110, 111

Simson, P. G., 181
Siniscalco, M., 107
Sivam, S. P., 211
Sivit, C., 195
Sjogren, B., 92
Skinner, R., 149, 160, 161, 162, 163
Skolnick, M., 61, 108
Slater, E., 15, 149
Slaugenhaulst, S. A., 109, 111
Small, J. G., 124, 130, 139
Smeal, T., 200, 210
Smeraldi, E., 6, 9
Smith, C., 14
Smith, D. R., 211
Smith, H., 50
Snyder, K. S., 129, 130
Snyder, S. H., 198
Sobol, S., 207, 208
Sonnenberg, J. L., 208
Sorensen, S., 188
Southern, E. M., 82
Spence, M. A., 94, 98
Spencer, R., 210
Spenec, A., 29
Spiegalman, B. M., 201
Spiegel, A. M., 196, 199
Spielberger, C. D., 105
Spitzer, R. L., 43, 159
Spitzer, R., 73
Spowart, G., 109
Srole, L., 7
St. Clair, D., 92, 109
Stabenau, J. R., 15
Stallone, F., 153
Stancer, H. C., 106, 123
Stanley, M., 184, 205
Starace, F., 143
Stein, L., 207
Sternberg, D. E., 212
Stewart, M. A., 197
Stockmeier, C. A., 187
Strober, M., 124, 125
Strunk, C., 211
Suarez, B. K., 93, 106
Sulser, F., 185, 187
Sun, Y. L., 200, 210
Sussex, J. N., 33, 73, 78, 83, 92, 101, 109, 149
Swanson, J. M., 17

Author Index

Taghavi, Z., 198
Takahashi, J. S., 204
Takeuchi, K., 211
Tanna, V. L., 106, 108, 109, 111
Tanzi, R. E., 65
Targum, S. D., 10, 31, 106, 149, 150, 151, 152, 155, 156, 157, 161, 163, 164, 166
Tatemoto, K., 207
Tauson, V. B., 124, 130, 139
Teich, N. M., 201
Teyssier, J. R., 110
Thase, M. E., 128
Theillie, A., 105
Thompson, W. D., 6, 10
Thoren, P., 181
Tideman, S., 94, 98
Tijan, R., 201
Tischler, A. S., 210, 211
Tischler, G. L., 152
Todd, R., 109
Toele, T. R., 204
Tohen, M., 126, 139
Tondo, L., 126
Toomey, K. E., 110
Torgersen, S., 15
Totoescu, A., 140
Traskman, L., 181
Trautner, E. M., 194
Troughton, E., 18
Trzebiatowska-Trzeciak, O., 9
Tsuang, M. T., 4, 5, 6, 8, 10, 14, 22, 120, 121, 123, 127, 146, 148, 149, 150, 151, 152, 153, 155, 157, 158, 159, 161, 162, 164, 165, 168
Tsui, L.-C., 46, 65
Turner, J. W., 107
Turner, W. J., 149

van Broeckhoven, C., 109
Van Calker, D., 203
Van Eerdewegh, M., 7, 31, 32, 101, 106, 123, 153
Van Eerdewegh, P., 107
van Houten, P., 181
Van Nguyen, T., 207
Van Praag, H. M., 66, 106
Vandermey, R., 127
Vartanian, F., 107
Vassart, G. P., 110
Vassart, G., 92
Vaughan, P. W., 128
Vaughn, C. E., 129, 130
Verma, I. M., 200, 201, 211
Virkkunen, M., 181
Visvader, J., 201
Vogel, F., 162
Vogt, P. K., 201
Volonte, C., 203
Voss, C. B., 124, 130, 139

Wagener, D. K., 123
Wahlestedt, C., 207
Wahlestedt, L., 207, 212
Walkers, M., 109
Wallace, M. R., 65
Warner, V., 121
Wasmuth, J., 92
Watkins, P. C., 65
Watson, J. D., 48
Watson, S., 121, 183
Weinberg, F., 17
Weinberger, C., 212
Weis, P., 124
Weiss, J. M., 178, 179, 181
Weiss, S. R. B., 124
Weissman, M. M., 6, 7, 10, 120, 121, 128, 129, 130, 152
Weitkamp, L. R., 106
Welner, A., 145
Welner, Z., 145
Wender, P. H., 18, 119, 121
Wesner, R. B., 109, 111
West, A., 146, 149, 169
Wetterburg, L., 92
Wexler, N., 65, 169
White, B. D., 208
White, R. L., 61, 108
Whybrow, P., 108
Wickramaratne, P., 121
Widerlov, E., 207, 212
Wikler, M., 147
Willey, C., 210
Williams, J. B. W., 43
Wilmotte, J., 107
Wilson, A. F., 111
Wilson, E., 108

Wing J. K., 140
Winokur, G., 10, 43, 106, 108, 109, 111
Wirtkamp, L. R., 106
Wolkowitz, O. M., 209
Worley, P. F., 198
Wraters, B., 109
Wright, A., 92
Wright, G., 181, 182, 209

Yagnow, R. L., 106
Yamamoto, K. R., 200, 210, 211
Yang, H. Y. T., 207, 208
Yang, N., 200, 211
Yang-Yen, H. F., 200, 210

Yoshinaga, S. K., 200, 210, 211
Yound, A. B., 65
Young, E. A., 183
Young, W. S., 212
Yuan, R., 50

Zahn-Waxler, C., 122, 154
Zarifian, E., 109
Zieglegansberger, W., 204
Ziff, E. B., 201
Zis, A. P., 126
Zohar, J., 205
Zsiga, M., 46, 65
Zubenko, G. S., 109, 111

Subject Index

Adenine (A), 48
Adenosine deaminase (ADA) deficiency, 46
Adolescent-onset:
  influence on, 123–124
  mood disorders and, 153
Adoption studies, genetic and environmental factors, 16–17
Adrenalectomy, 209
Aftercare, 126
Age-period interaction, 7–8
Alleles, 56–57, 91–92
Aminobutyric acid (GABA), 182
Amish, study of Old Order:
  chromosome 11, 82–84, 109
  diagnosis, reliability of, 73
  epidemiologic basis of, 73–76
  follow-up, 73, 84
  genetic linkage, DNA methods, 82–83
  heterogeneity, 160
  inbreeding, 162
  inheritance patterns, 77–82
  linkage study, 76–77
  markers, 87–89
  maternal influences, 122–123, 154
  objectives, 70–71
  pedigree 110:
    bipolar affective disorder and, 84–86
    extensions to, 86
  pedigree 210, 86–87
  replication, 83–87
  requisites for, 71–73
Anger dyscontrol, 43
Animal models:
  development of, 177–178
  genetic vulnerability studies, 187–190
  learned helplessness in, 178–179

melancholia, neurochemical anatomy of, 180–187
  psychotropic drug treatments, effect of, 179–180
Ankylosing spondylitis, 57
Antidepressants:
  animal model studies, effect of, 179
  response to, 153
  treatment strategy, 126, 139
Antipsychotics, animal studies of, 180
Anxiety neurosis, genetic factors, 15
AP-1, 201
Artistic creativity, 43
Assortative mating, 15, 149, 161
Attention-deficit disorder:
  adoption studies of, 17
  bipolar spectrum, 150

B-adrenergic receptors (B-AR):
  animal studies of, 180, 184–185
  RFLP analysis and, 65–66
Benzodiazepines, animal studies of, 180
Biological Psychiatry Collaborative Program, World Health Organization, 106
Bipolar disorder:
  Amish, 74–75, 78–79
  bipolar spectrum and, 150
  diagnostic hierarchies, 36, 38
  environmental factors and, 152
  epidemiologic studies of, 5–6
  family studies of, 9–10
  gender and, 152
  with hypomania, 32–33
  inheritance patterns, 79, 152
  onset of, 153
  relapse, 130

Subject Index

relative risk for, 121
twin studies, concordance rate, 13–14, 23, 151
Bipolar I disorder:
  defined, 23
  vegetative symptoms, 33
Bipolar II disorder:
  Amish, 75
  classification of, 33
  defined, 32
  empirical risk data, 150
  vegetative symptoms, 33
Bipolar manic-depressive illness, color blindness and, 106
Bipolar schizoaffective disorder, 32
Bipolar spectrum, 150
Birth cohort effect, 7
Bradykinin, 203
Burden of illness, genetic counseling and, 162–163
Butyrophenones, animal studies of, 180

Calmodulin kinase, 203
Carbachol, 203
Catecholamine hypothesis, 194
Chromatin, 49
Chromosome 11:
  Amish, 82–84, 109
  linkage to, 101
Chromosome 4, RFLP marker on, 65
Chromosome 7, RFLP marker on, 65
Chromosome 6, 106
Chromosome X, 107, 110–112
Chronic hypomania, 101
Chronicity, rate of, 125
Clinical assessment:
  age at, 161
  implications for, 124–125
Clinical interview:
  Amish, 74
  family studies, 10
  genetic counseling, 158–159
  guides for, 40–41
  Orthodox Jewish community, 158–159
Clinicians, experienced, 39–40
Cloning strategies, 52, 55
Codon, 49

Color blindness:
  Amish, 76
  classical markers, 106
  as polymorphism, 56
Community mental health movement, 126
Complementary DNA (cDNA), 52–53
Concordant twins, 12
Confidentiality, 131, 169
Consanguinity, 162
Coriell Institute for Medical Research (CIMR), 84
Corticotropin releasing factor (CRF), animal study of, 182–183
Cosegregation, 91–92
Cross-fostering studies, 16, 18
Cyclic adenosine monophosphate (cAMP), 199
Cyclothymia, 35, 159
Cystic fibrosis, 65
Cytosine (C), 48

Danish Psychiatric Twin Register, 13, 18
Deoxyribonucleic acid (DNA), *see* DNA
Depression, maternal, effect of, 122
Depressive neurosis, genetic factors, 15
Dexamethasone suppression test, 183
Diagnostic and Statistical Manual Mental Disorders (DSM-III, DSM-III Revised), 43
Diagnostic hierarchies:
  alternative to, 38–39
  utilization of, 36, 38
Diagnostic Interview for Genetic Studies (DIGS), 43
Diagnosticians, "best-estimate consensus," 41–42
Disclosure, 168–169
Dizygotic twins:
  concordance rate, 151
  genetic and environmental studies, 12–16
DNA:
  basic recombinant, 50, 52, 83
  library, creation of, 52–53, 55
  replication, 48
  structure of, 47–49
DNA molecular markers, 108–111
Dopamine-2 receptor gene (D2), as genetic marker, 109

Subject Index

Double helix, 48
Dual mating, 161, 166
Dysthymia, 159

Eating disorders, 150
EcoR1, 62
Educational workshops, family psychoeducational approach, 130
Environmental factors:
   family studies and, 11–12. *See also* Twin studies
   significance of, 3
   types of, 122
Ethics, 169

Family conflict, effect of, 130
Family History-Research Diagnostic Criteria (FH-RDC), 43
Family Interview for Genetic Studies (FIGS), 43
Family pedigree linkage analysis method, 93
First-degree relatives, genetic risk for, 4, 23, 107, 120, 151
5-HT reuptake system, animal studies of, 181, 184–185
Flanking markers, 64
Fluoxetine, animal studies of, 180, 185
Fluvoxamine, animal studies of, 186
Fornix, role of, 182
fos gene expression:
   cultured neuronal cells, 201–204
   in rat brain, 204–206
Fragile X syndrome, 110

Gametes, 92
Gene amplification, polymerase chain reaction (PCR) and, 108
Gene expression:
   fos, 201–206
   glucocorticoids (GC), 208–210, 212
   lithium and, 201–211
   second messenger-mediated, 199–201
Gene mapping, 61, 67, 75
Gene of interest, isolation of, 64–65
Gene therapy, history of, 46
Genetic counseling:
   diagnosis, establishment of, 158–161
   fears and concerns, addressing, 164–168

follow-up, 161, 168
generally, 146, 155–156
genetic information, communicating, 163–164
illness, effect on, 162–163
motive assessment, 156–158
pedigree risk, 161–162
psychoeducational approach and, 138–139
Genetic counselor, role of, 155–168
Genetic linkage:
   defined, 91
   detection methods, 93–98
   limitations of, 98–102
   success of, 92
Genetic models:
   limited loci polygenic (LLP) model, 20
   multifactorial polygenic (MFP) model, 20
   single major locus (SML) model, 19–20
Genetics, defined, 3
Genomic libraries, creation of, 52–53, 55
Glucocorticoids (GC), gene expression and, 208–210, 212
Glucose 6-phosphate dehydrogenase (G6PD), 56, 107
G proteins, lithium and, 198–199
Growth factors, lithium and, 195, 212
Guanine (G), 48
Guanine triphosphate (GTP), 198

Haplotypes, 57
Harvey-ras (HRAS), as genetic marker, 83, 86, 109
Hasidic Jewish community, consanguinity and, 162
Heterogeneity, linkage studies, 107, 109
Hippocampus, role of, 180, 182
Histones, 49
Hormones, lithium and, 195, 212
Human Genome Project, 67
Human leukocyte antigen (HLA):
   Amish, 76–77
   defined, 57
   linkage studies, 106
Huntington's Disease, 65, 169
Hybridization, 50, 53
Hypomania, early manifestation of, 31

Subject Index 233

Hypothalamic-pituitary axis (HPA), animal studies of, 181-184
Hypothalamus, receptor function and, 180

Imipramine, animal studies of, 185
Independent assortment, 106
Inositol depletion hypothesis, 197-198, 211
Insulin (INS), as genetic marker, 83, 86, 109
Interviewer blindness, purpose of, 8, 39, 41, 74, 83

Junk DNA, 60

Kraepelin concept, 13

Labile personality, 35
Learned helplessness, see Animal models, learned helplessness in
Liability, distribution of, 20-21
Ligands, lithium and, 195-196
Ligases, 52
Limited loci polygenic (LLP) genetic model, 20
Linkage analysis:
   basics of, 55-57, 59
   classical markers, 105-108
   DNA molecular markers, 108-111
   family pedigree method, 93-94
   gene transmission model, 188
   heterozygosity and, 62
   history of, 46-47
   misclassification and, 98-100
   pedigrees and, 60
   replication and, 101
   sib-pair method, 93
   success of, 102
LIPED:
   development of, 94
   modified version of, 98
Lithium:
   action site, theories of, 194
   antidepressant action of, 212
   fos expression, in rat brain, 204-206
   gene expression:
      cultured neuronal cells, 201-204
      neuropeptide, 206-211

      in rat brain, 204-206
   second messenger-mediated, 199-201
   G proteins, effect on, 198-199
   half-life, 212
   history of, 194
   inositol depletion hypothesis, 197-198, 211
   interpersonal problems and, 129
   phosphoinositide pathway and, 197-198
   preventive treatment and, 126
   response to, 153-154
   signal transduction, 195-197
   as treatment strategy, 127
Lod scores, calculation of, 95-97

Major depression:
   Amish, 74
   risk for, 7, 121, 123
   treatment strategies, 139
Mania, cholinergic hypothesis of, 66
Manic-depressive psychoses:
   B-adrenergic receptors (B-AR) gene and, 66
   c-Harvey-ras-A (HRAS) and, 109
   epidemiologic studies of, 5-6
   family studies, 8-9
Marital conflict, effect of, 130
Maternal influence, as environmental factor, 122-123, 154
Meiosis, 57
Melancholia, neurochemical anatomy of, 180-187
Mendelian inheritance rules, mood disorders and, 19-20
Mental status assessment, genetic counseling and, 163
Messenger RNA (mRNA):
   conversion to, 49
   enk, 208
   fos, 202, 207
   gene expression and, 199-201
Mianserin, animal studies of, 180
Minor depressive disorder, 34-35, 101
Misclassification, significance of, 35-36, 98-99, 124-125
Monoamine oxidase inhibitors (MAOIs), animal model studies of, 179

Subject Index

Monozygotic twins:
  concordance rate, 151, 153
  genetic and environmental studies, 12–16
Mood disorders:
  adoption studies, 17–18, 120
  empirical risk for, 152
  environmental factors and, 153
  family, effect on, 128–131
  family studies:
    epidemiologic population studies, 5–8
    genetic hypothesis, 4–5
    interpretation of, 5, 120
  generational impact of, 121–124
  genetic transmission, mode determination, 19–23
  incidence of, 127
  onset, age of, 153
  Orthodox Jewish community, see Orthodox Jewish community, mood disorders in
  twin studies, 14–15, 23, 120
Multifactorial polygenic (MFP) genetic model, 20–21
Mutations, 49, 60
Myoinositol 1-phosphatase (M1P), 197, 203

National Institute of General Medical Science (NIGMS), *Cell Repository Catalog*, 84
National Institute of Mental Health (NIHM):
  Clinical Neuroscience Branch, Intramural Research Program (IRP), 88
  Collaborative Study of Depression, 10
  Diagnostic Centers for Psychiatric Linkage Studies, 43
  diagnostic procedures, 43
  Project DART (Depression Awareness and Recognition Training), 139
Nerve growth factor, 203
Neuropeptide gene expression, lithium and, 206–211
Neuropeptide Y (NPY):
  gene expression, 200, 207–208, 210
  mood disorders and, 207

Neurotransmitters, lithium and, 195
Nucleotide bases:
  base pairing, 48
  defined, 47
  list of, 48

Obsessive-compulsive disorder, 150
Odds ratio, 94
Offspring, risk for:
  environmental, 122, 154
  genetic, 121, 139
Old Order Amish, see Amish, study of Old Order
Onset:
  age of, 123, 152–153
  new, 101
Orthodox Jewish community:
  disclosure, 168
  divorce and, 163
  family planning, 166
  generally, 147–148
  genetic counseling:
    burden of illness, 163
    case example, 167–168
    follow-up, 168
    motivation for, 157–158
    pedigree risk, 161–162
    rabbi, role in, 157–158, 166–167
  mood disorders in:
    age of onset, 152–153
    bipolar spectrum, 150
    empirical risk data, 150–152
    environmental factors, 153–155
    gender, 152–153
    incomplete penetrance, 149–150
    inheritance mode, 148–149
    pharmacogenetics, 153
    stigmatization, 147–148, 158, 165

Panic disorder, 150
Pedigree assessment:
  diagnostic data, procedures for, 39–41
  diagnostic evaluations:
    criteria selection, 42
    guidelines for, 41–42
    procedures, 42–44
  disorders:
    groupings of, 35–36, 38

Subject Index

selection of, 30–32
types of, 32–35
family selection, diagnostic criteria, 29–30
laboratory tests, lack of, 28, 31
Pedigree segregation analysis:
defined, 19
multifactorial polygenic (MFP) genetic model, 21
single major locus (SML) genetic model, 20
Penetrance, 94, 98, 149–150
Phase, uncertainty of, 96
Phenothiazines, animal studies of, 180
Phorbol 12-myristate 13-acetate (PMA), 20
Phosphoinositide pathway, 197–198
pi106-aminobutyric acid (GABA) receptor (GABRA), 110
PKC, 201, 203–204
Plasmids, 52
Polygenic inheritance, 20
Polymorphism, 56–57, 61, 67
Prednisone, study of, 208
Prevalence analysis, 19
Proband, defined, 4, 138
Progenitor Trace Study, Amish, 79, 81
Project DART (Depression Awareness and Recognition Training), 139
Psychoeducational approach:
case studies, 133–138
description of, 131–132
effect of, 130–131
family environment and, 128
genetic counseling and, 138–139
goals, 132–133
purpose of, generally, 128, 131

Recombinant DNA era, 46, 60
Recombination, 57
Refractory rapid cycling disorder, 163
Relapse:
bipolar disorder, 130
noncompliance and, 127
prevention of, 126, 128
rate of, 111, 125, 130
schizophrenia, 129
Research Diagnostic Criteria (RDC), 43, 73

Restriction endonucleases:
location sites, 60
recombinant DNA and, 50, 61
Restriction fragment length polymorphisms (RFLP) analysis:
candidate gene approach, 65–66
defined, 61
process, 60–62, 64–65
RNA, messenger(mRNA), see Messenger RNA (mRNA)

Schedule for Affective Disorders and Schizophrenia (SADS-LB), 43, 158
Schizophrenia:
adoption study, 119
Amish, 125
misdiagnosis of, 124–125
pathogenesis of, 193
relapse, 129
trait-dependent marker of, 66
Second-degree relatives, genetic risk for, 152
Sedative, animal studies of, 180
Segregation analyses, Amish, 77–78
Selective breeding, 188
Sib-pair linkage analysis method, 93, 96
Siblings, risk for, 152
Sibships, 85
Sickle cell anemia, 49
Single major locus (SML) genetic model, 19–20
Sleep-wake cycle, disruption of, 154
Southern blotting, 61
Stigmatization:
Amish, 83
effects of, 127
Orthodox Jewish community, 147–148, 158, 165
Structured Clinical Interview for Diagnosis (SCID), 43
Subtraction libraries, 190
Suicide:
B-adrenergic receptors (B-AR) and, 184
incidence of, 125
risk for, 121
serotonin levels and, 181
u-receptors and, 188–189

Therapeutic relationship, 155, 160
Thymine (T), 48
Transmission modes:
  father-to-son, 79, 149, 152
  linkage analysis and, 188
  mood disorders, 19–23, 148–149
  mother-to-son, 152
Trazadone, animal studies of, 180, 186
Treatment:
  implications for, 124–125
  strategies for, 125–128
Trinucleotide repeats, 88
Tumor-promoter-responsive (TRE) DNA elements, 201
Twin studies:
  concordance rate, 12–13, 151, 153
  family aggregation, 31
  genetic and environmental factors, 12–16

Tyrosine hydroxylase (TH), as genetic marker, 109

U937 cells, 203
Unipolar depressive disorder, 33–34
Unipolar disorder:
  adolescent-onset, 124
  Amish, 74–75
  bipolar spectrum and, 150
  environmental factors and, 152
  family studies of, 9–10
  risk for, 6–8, 11, 121
  treatment strategy, 139
  twin studies, 23, 151
Unipolar schizoaffective disorder, 34

Variability in the length of tandem repetitive DNA elements (VNTR), 61